The 2001 Outbreak of Foot and Mouth Disease

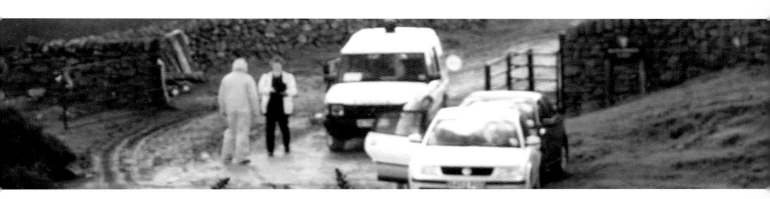

REPORT BY THE COMPTROLLER AND AUDITOR GENERAL
HC 939 Session 2001-2002: 21 June 2002

LONDON: The Stationery Office
£17.75

Ordered by the
House of Commons
to be printed on 18 June 2002

This report has been prepared under Section 6 of the
National Audit Act 1983 for presentation to the House
of Commons in accordance with Section 9 of the Act.

John Bourn   **National Audit Office**
Comptroller and Auditor General   **14 June 2002**

The National Audit Office study team consisted of:

Richard Eales, Pamela Thomas, David Bostock,
Stewart Lingard, Ian Derbyshire, Allison Burmiston
and Howard Kitson

This report can be found on the National Audit Office
web site at www.nao.gov.uk

**For further information about the National Audit Office
please contact:**

National Audit Office
Press Office
157-197 Buckingham Palace Road
Victoria
London
SW1W 9SP

Tel: 020 7798 7400

Email: enquiries@nao.gsi.gov.uk

Contents

© Photographs appearing on pages 5,8,10,11,21,50,51,55,59,67,74,76,86,88,90,101and 131 courtesy of PA Photos.

executive summary

1   Foot and mouth disease was suspected at an abattoir in Essex on 19 February 2001 and confirmed the following day. By the time the disease had been eradicated in September 2001, more than six million animals had been slaughtered: over four million for disease control purposes; and over two million for welfare reasons. The direct cost to the public sector is estimated at over £3 billion and the cost to the private sector is estimated at over £5 billion.

2   At least 57 farms had already been infected with the virus when the disease was confirmed on 20 February 2001. The disease spread quickly and there were outbreaks in 44 counties, unitary authorities and metropolitan districts and over 2,000 premises were infected **(Figure 1)**. The scale and impact of the epidemic were immense: greater than that of the last serious outbreak in Britain, in 1967-68. In mid-April 2001, at the height of the crisis, more than 10,000 vets, soldiers, field and support staff, assisted by thousands more working for contractors, were engaged in fighting the disease. Up to 100,000 animals were slaughtered and disposed of each day in what was a massive and complex logistical operation. Tourism suffered the largest financial impact from the outbreak, with visitors to Britain and the countryside deterred by the initial blanket closure of footpaths by local authorities and media images of mass pyres.

3   The epidemic lasted for 32 weeks, the last case being confirmed on 30 September 2001 on a farm near Appleby in Cumbria. On 22 January 2002 the United Kingdom was re-instated on the OIE[1]-list of countries free of foot and mouth disease, and on 5 February 2002 the European Commission lifted remaining meat and animal export restrictions.

4   Compensation and other payments to farmers are expected to total nearly £1.4 billion. Direct costs of measures to deal with the epidemic including the purchase of goods and services to eradicate the disease are expected to amount to nearly £1.3 billion. Other public sector costs are estimated at £0.3 billion. In the private sector, the areas most affected by the outbreak were agriculture, the food chain and supporting services, which incurred net costs of £0.6 billion; and tourism and supporting industries, which lost revenues of between £4.5 billion and £5.4 billion. The Treasury has estimated that the net economic effect of the outbreak was less than 0.2 per cent of gross domestic product[2] (this would be equivalent to less than £2 billion).

1   Counties with cases of foot and mouth disease

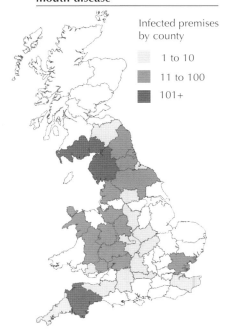

Infected premises by county

1 to 10

11 to 100

101+

Source: Department for the Environment, Food and Rural Affairs

---

1   The Office Internationale des Epizooties, with 158 member countries, sets sanitary rules for international trade in animals and animal products and disseminates veterinary scientific information on animal disease control.

2   The net economic effect was less than the £5 billion cost to agriculture and tourism because many of the losses suffered by individuals and firms led to equivalent amounts being spent elsewhere in the economy.

5   The Department for Environment, Food and Rural Affairs (formerly the Ministry of Agriculture, Fisheries and Food) (the Department[3]) took the lead in dealing with the outbreak. Many other departments and agencies were also involved and farmers, private contractors and voluntary and stakeholder groups played important roles. From the outset the Prime Minister and Cabinet were closely engaged, receiving regular briefings on the developing situation and the progress made in controlling the disease. The Government's priority was to combat the disease with whatever resources were needed. The Government's view was that best value for money would be obtained by stamping the disease out quickly.

6   Under the Scotland Act of 1998, legislation on all animal health matters has been devolved to the Scottish Parliament and policy development and implementation made the responsibility of Scottish Ministers. During the 2001 outbreak, Scottish Ministers operated within an agreed policy framework whilst taking account of local circumstances.

7   Some, but not all, animal health functions were transferred to the National Assembly for Wales in 1999, but the operational 'on the ground' disease control functions in the Animal Health Act 1981 and the Foot and Mouth Disease Order 1983 continued as functions of the Department post-devolution. Under the Animal Health Act 1981, the National Assembly for Wales makes secondary legislation jointly with the Department and makes regulations under section 2(2) of the European Communities Act 1972, mainly to implement Community decisions on import and export of animal carcasses and animal products. During the 2001 outbreak decisions affecting Wales were in practice taken by the Department in consultation with the National Assembly.

Scope of our examination

8   Against the above background, we examined the adequacy of contingency planning for an outbreak of foot and mouth disease, how quickly and effectively the disease was eradicated and the cost-effectiveness of the action taken. The investigation covered England, Scotland and Wales. It did not cover Northern Ireland, which has its own animal health legislation and veterinary service.

---

3   The "Department" is used in this report to describe the Ministry of Agriculture, Fisheries and Food, which became part of the Department for Environment, Food and Rural Affairs in June 2001.

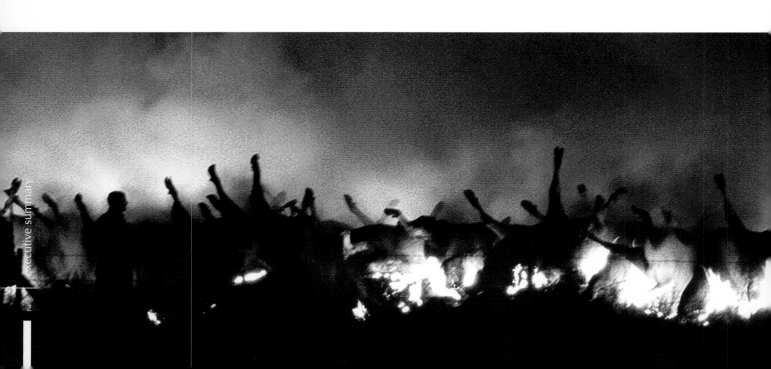

executive summary

2

Our main conclusions

Preparing for a possible outbreak of foot and mouth disease (Part 2 of the Report)

9 We found that:

a **The nature and scale of the 2001 outbreak were unprecedented**. The source case, on a pig farm, was discovered two days after foot and mouth disease was confirmed to be in Britain. However, it was apparent that the premises had probably been infected for several weeks. The main transmitters of the virus were sheep, where identification of the clinical signs of disease was particularly difficult. And the outbreak occurred at a time of year when large numbers of sheep were being marketed and moved. Consequently, the disease was already widely 'seeded' across the country by the time the first case was detected. The Department believes that given the unprecedented nature of what happened it is unrealistic to expect any contingency planning to have fully prepared it for the chain of events that occurred. Senior veterinary officers in other countries and the European Commissioner for Health and Consumer Protection have commented that the nature and magnitude of the events in Britain were such that any country would have struggled under the circumstances. Many countries are revising their contingency arrangements in the light of Britain's experience in 2001.

b **The Department had prepared contingency plans which met European Union requirements**. The plans comprised a national contingency plan for Great Britain; local contingency plans; and standing field instructions for veterinary and other staff on the practical measures to be taken in the event of an outbreak. The plans were approved by the European Commission in 1993 and had been updated in various ways since then. In the event, contingency plans worked in those areas where there were relatively few cases. In the worst hit areas, the disease had spread widely before it had been identified. The unprecedented scale of the outbreaks in these areas meant that the resources needed to deal with the disease rapidly went beyond what had been envisaged in the contingency plans.

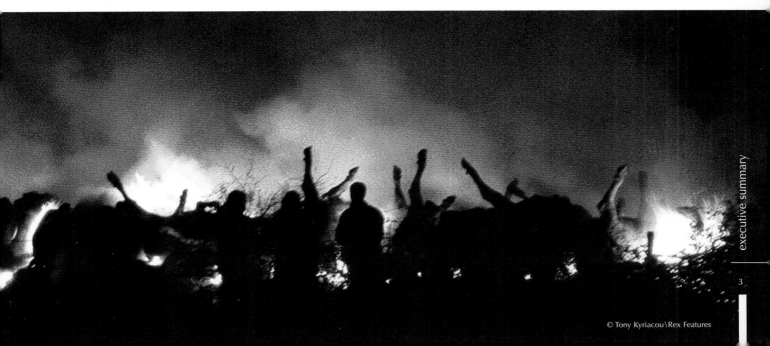

c   **The Department's contingency plans were not sufficient to deal with an outbreak on this scale (Figure 2)**. It is unrealistic to expect that any contingency plan could have coped with all the problems and difficulties that arose or that the Department could have forecast the unprecedented nature of the 2001 outbreak. Nevertheless, more thorough contingency planning would allow the Department to be better prepared for a future outbreak. During the course of the epidemic the Department responded to gaps and limitations in its plans in an active and innovative manner.

d   **Following eradication of the disease, the Department is revising its contingency plans (Figure 3)**. The Department is also working to revise and update existing local plans and veterinary guidance and to codify the experience gained from the 2001 outbreak into interim operational plans. The plans will be revised, amended and developed as necessary in the light of the recommendations of the Independent Inquiries announced by the Government into the 2001 outbreak of foot and mouth disease. Similar work is under way in Scotland and Wales.

2   The Department's contingency plans were not sufficient to deal with an outbreak on the scale of that in 2001

There are lessons to be learned from the 2001 outbreak to help the Department in preparing contingency plans against any future outbreak. Some of the key lessons are set out below.

The implications of vaccination could have been more fully considered. Routine vaccination of livestock to prevent or slow foot and mouth disease is not legal in the European Union. European Union law permits the use of emergency vaccination only as part of a stamping out policy where appropriate. Before the outbreak the Department had drawn up detailed instructions for the use of emergency vaccination but did not distribute these to local offices because it considered that any vaccination programme would have to be co-ordinated and resourced nationally and would need the detailed agreement of the European Commission. At the height of the outbreak the Government accepted that there might be a case for a limited emergency vaccination programme and the Department began to draw up plans to vaccinate cattle in Cumbria and Dumfries and Galloway and possibly Devon. The necessary support of farmers, veterinarians, retailers and food manufacturers was not forthcoming, however, and vaccination did not go ahead.

The plans were based on the most likely scenario and other scenarios were not considered. In line with European Commission guidance, the Department's plans were based on the supposition that there would not be more than 10 infected premises at any one time. The Department considered this to be a sensible basis for planning as most outbreaks in Europe during the 1990s suggested that the most likely scenario would involve only a small number of infected premises at the outset. International scientific advice was that the risk of foot and mouth disease being introduced to the United Kingdom was low. The Department believes that, had there been only 10 infected premises in 2001, its contingency plans would have worked. The plans did work in those areas where there were relatively few cases. In the event, however, at least 57 premises were infected before the initial diagnosis was made. A consequence of not considering other scenarios was that little prior consideration had been given to the impact on non-farming businesses that a large-scale epidemic might have and what the economic costs might be.

Recommendations from previous animal health reports had largely been adopted with the exception of some recommendations from an internal report in 1999. The Department's contingency plans incorporated most of the recommendations made in the **Northumberland report** on the 1967-68 outbreak of foot and mouth disease. We examined four instances where it did not appear that the Department had fully followed the Northumberland report's recommendations. The Department told us that, 30 years on from the report, its plans for dealing with an outbreak had been modified to some degree compared to the 1969 report's recommendations. The Department considers that it had implemented the Northumberland report's recommendations in all material respects. In 1998-99 the **Drummond report** on preparedness across the State Veterinary Service found considerable variations in the Service's readiness to deal with outbreaks of exotic notifiable diseases, including foot and mouth. Existing contingency plans in many areas had not been updated because of other priorities and limited staff resources. The Drummond report expressed concern that a rapid spread of foot and mouth disease could quickly overwhelm the State Veterinary Service's resources, particularly if a number of separate outbreaks occurred at the same time. By July 2000 the Department had made progress on many of the action areas but implementation of other key issues was delayed by the need to attend to other high priority work.

Stakeholders were not formally consulted in preparing contingency plans. Tackling a serious outbreak of animal disease requires effective co-operation among a number of government departments, including those responsible for the environment, public health, transport, the armed services, the countryside and tourism. Any strategy for dealing with the disease and its wider impacts also depends for its success on the active co-operation of those closely affected. However, in preparing the national contingency plan and the veterinary instructions for foot and mouth disease, the Department had not formally consulted other key stakeholders, such as other government departments, local authorities and representatives of farmers and the veterinary profession. Some stakeholders had nevertheless been involved in simulation exercises as part of local contingency planning.

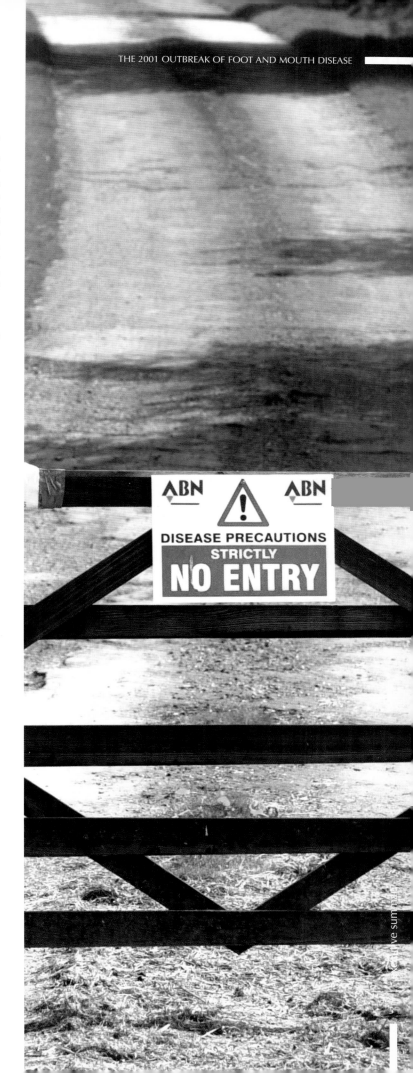

3 **The Department's interim national contingency plan for foot and mouth disease**

The interim contingency plan does not seek to pre-empt the results of official inquiries and will be reviewed once their findings have been made public. The plan codifies lessons learned during the 2001 foot and mouth outbreak. It is a temporary measure, dealing solely with operational issues. The current Great Britain foot and mouth contingency plan has been in existence for many years and has been regularly updated. The plan was approved by the European Commission in 1993. The interim contingency plan was presented for discussion on 12 March 2002 and placed on the Department's website. A consultative meeting with stakeholders took place on the same day and another on 20 March 2002.

Details of the plan

1   The plan is split into sections outlining structures, lines of communication, roles and responsibilities at both national and local levels.

2   An alert system is outlined describing actions that need to be taken upon report of a suspected case (amber alert) and upon confirmation of disease (red alert).

3   The response to the disease alert would be controlled using the recognised Gold, Silver and Bronze Command structure (Gold - Strategic, Silver - Tactical, Bronze - Operational).

4   At a national level there is consideration of the role of a Joint Co-ordination Centre, a Disease Emergency Control Centre, a Foot and Mouth Disease Programme Board and a Co-ordination Committee (or perhaps the Cabinet Office Briefing Room).

5   Use is made of a technique called process mapping to define initial action and responsibilities.

6   Further detail is provided on issues such as: resources, training, accommodation, information technology, procurement, stores, disposal, serology, financial, accounting and management information, communications, publicity and disease awareness, stakeholder involvement, vaccination, health and safety, and contingency testing.

7   The plan provides job descriptions for key personnel (such as Regional Operations Directors) at both national and local levels.

8   Further information provides detail on the relationship with the devolved administrations at an operational level, personal biosecurity protocols, transport specifications, daily situation reports, key personnel contacts, and foot and mouth stock lists held at Animal Health Offices.

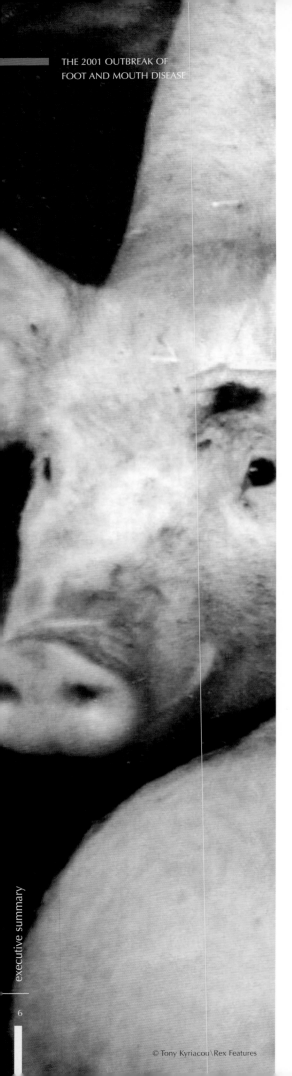

© Tony Kyriacou\Rex Features

executive summary

Handling the outbreak (Part 3 of the Report)

10 We found that:

a   **Foot and mouth disease was eradicated quickly in some areas**. In the Infected Areas covered by half of the 18 Disease Control Centres, the time between confirmation of the first and last infected premises was two months or less. The Department also had a number of successes in preventing the further spread of the disease (**Figure 4**). The disease was eradicated in seven months, the same time that it took to deal with the smaller outbreak in 1967-68.

b   **Those involved worked extremely hard to bring the epidemic under control**. The disease was eradicated through the commitment and dedication of the Department's staff and many others who assisted in the disease control campaign. Those in the field worked punishingly long days in stressful and often distressing conditions. Administrative staff also worked hard, often in cramped and temporary accommodation. Those from other parts of government, the voluntary sector, farmers and contractors also made a substantial contribution.

c   **There were severe problems in handling the outbreak in the worst-hit areas**. The widespread 'seeding' of the virus before it was discovered and the rapid spread of the disease quickly stretched the Department's resources. Consequently, during the early weeks of the crisis, there were delays in identification, slaughter and disposal of infected and exposed animals. As the outbreak progressed and experience was gained on the ground, the Department developed new control measures to deal with the difficulties that arose. Some of the problems faced by the Department and the measures taken to deal with them are illustrated in **Figure 5**.

---

4   **Successes in preventing the further spread of foot and mouth disease in 2001**

The Department successfully contained the outbreak substantially to those areas initially infected with the disease, thereby protecting large areas of important livestock production in adjoining and more distant areas.

The disease was kept out of much of East Anglia, the East Midlands, southern England, west Wales and central and northern Scotland. This protected important dairying and pig industry areas. The outbreak would probably have been much more extensive if the disease had been allowed to spread to the pig areas, as pigs are major shedders of the virus.

By mid-April 2001 the disease had been stamped out in most parts of central and eastern England. Outbreaks were also brought quite quickly under control in Anglesey and southern Scotland.

The Department was also successful in ensuring that once the disease had been stamped out in an area it did not reappear. In 1967-68 the tail of the epidemic had been prolonged by a re-emergence of the disease during restocking of previously infected farms.

---

5   The nature and scale of the outbreak posed immense problems for the Department

Organisational structures improved as the crisis developed. Operations were initially directed by the Department's veterinary officers. But by mid-March 2001 the size of the outbreak was placing impossibly heavy demands on the State Veterinary Service and new structures were introduced. The Cabinet Office Briefing Room was opened, supported by a Joint Co-ordination Centre at the Department's headquarters, and senior administrators were appointed to the main Disease Control Centres as Regional Operations Directors. These new arrangements improved the response to the disease: state vets were given more time for veterinary work; resource bottlenecks, particularly those affecting slaughter and disposal, were eased; and measures were taken to promote cross-agency co-ordination and improve communications with stakeholders.

It took time to get other agencies involved. The scale and impact of the epidemic was so great that other government departments and agencies, local authorities, voluntary organisations and stakeholders inevitably became involved. They all had important contributions to make in helping to combat the disease. The armed services were kept informed from the outset and were involved in regular discussions with the Department. The Department decided not to call for substantial military assistance until three weeks after the start of the outbreak because the Government considered that the early stages of the epidemic presented no obvious requirement for military participation. The armed services went on to play a key supportive role, assisting centrally and locally in the organisational and logistical arrangements, particularly for slaughter, transport and disposal. The Department began liaising with other government departments, agencies and local authorities from day 1 of the outbreak, although some bodies felt that they could have been more directly involved earlier.

The Department overcame a severe shortage of vets. Vets played a key role in diagnosing disease, overseeing slaughter arrangements and providing advice to farmers and others. During the early weeks of the 2001 outbreak, there were too few vets and this delayed disease control. The Chief Veterinary Officer called on agreed standby arrangements nationally and internationally from 23 February 2001. Veterinary resources were built up and by mid-April 2001 the Department had the number of vets it felt were needed to contain the outbreak.

A national movement ban on 23 February 2001 prevented greater spread of the disease but with hindsight could have been imposed earlier in this outbreak. Preventing the movement of infected animals is a vital element of disease control since direct animal to animal contact is the quickest means of virus transmission. The Department imposed a local movement ban on 21 February 2001 around the first infected premises and supplier farms and a national movement ban (and closure of livestock markets) on 23 February 2001. These bans prevented greater geographical spread of the disease. The Department did not impose a national movement ban earlier because it believed that local movement controls would control the disease. A national ban would have been unprecedented and the Department considered that the epidemiological evidence at the time did not exist to justify a countrywide ban.

Because compliance with local control measures was incomplete they were not fully effective in stopping the spread of the disease. From the second week of the outbreak, the disease was chiefly being spread locally over distances of less than three kilometres. The Department believes that an important factor in this spread was poor compliance with biosecurity standards by some farmers. 'Restricted Infected Areas' were later established with much stricter biosecurity controls. These intensified arrangements were important in helping to bring the outbreak to an end.

The Department introduced a contiguous cull to help check the spread of the disease. This was hugely controversial. In mid-March 2001 the Government's scientific advisers provided evidence that, because the Department was initially having to "chase" the disease this could potentially lead to an exponential growth in the number of new cases. The Department responded by introducing a number of changes in approach, including the slaughter of susceptible animals on premises contiguous to infected premises. These changes helped to control the disease but led to the culling of many animals that may have been exposed but were not showing clinical signs of the disease. The contiguous cull met considerable resistance from some farmers and others. The Department considers that the cull saved many animal lives by preventing animals from becoming infected with the disease.

The Department was unable in some cases to achieve the rapid slaughter of infected or exposed animals. Animals identified as being infected or at risk need to be slaughtered quickly to check the spread of the disease. However, in the early weeks the Department was unable to achieve rapid slaughter, mainly because of the shortage of vets. Performance improved from late March 2001 onwards.

There were huge logistical problems in disposing of millions of slaughtered animals. The backlog of slaughtered animals awaiting disposal built up to a peak of over 200,000 carcasses in early April 2001. The most commonly used methods of disposal were burning, rendering, landfill and burial. In practice the Department experienced problems with all the methods used. Many carcasses were disposed of in March 2001 on mass pyres. But this generated negative images in the media and had profound effects for the tourist industry. Some 1.3 million carcasses were disposed of at mass burial sites but public protests and technical problems prevented greater use of some sites. The Department considers that the problems with the various disposal options had not contributed to delays in slaughter.

Communications and information systems were severely stretched during the epidemic. The Department found it difficult in the crisis conditions to get its key instructions and messages across and to obtain good quality information from the field. At a national level, the Department engaged stakeholders positively from an early date. Locally, external communications were less satisfactory initially and on occasions the Department may not always have listened to local opinion. Local communications improved after Regional Operations Directors were appointed.

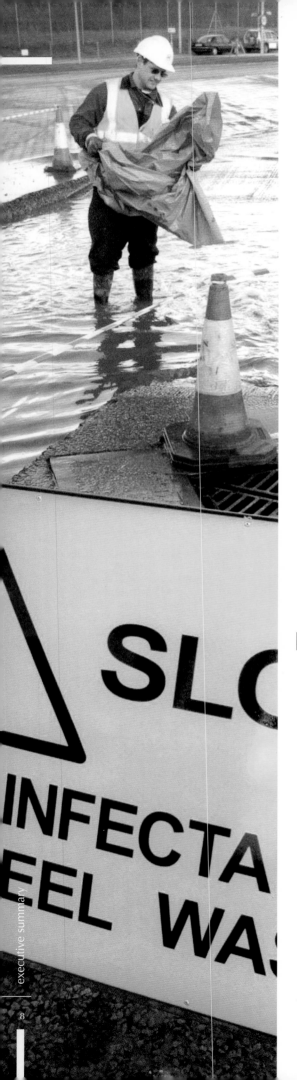

Controlling the costs of the outbreak (Part 4 of the Report)

11 We found that:

a **There were difficulties in administering the compensation and payment schemes to farmers.** Farmers received compensation for animals that were slaughtered for disease control purposes and payments for animals slaughtered under the Livestock Welfare (Disposal) Scheme. The sheer volume of cases put both schemes under enormous pressure and this led to costs being higher than they might otherwise have been in more normal circumstances (**Figure 6 opposite**).

b **The procurement of services and supplies was costly.** Large numbers of professional and administrative staff had to be brought together quickly and deployed across the country. A wide range of goods and services, many of them in short supply, had to be procured to meet urgent demands. Consequently systems of cost and financial control were put under great strain. The Department's negotiating position was weakened in many instances by the need to get things done quickly. After initial difficulties the Department took action to control costs.

c **Financial controls over payments were strengthened after initial problems.** Many of the Department's payment processes operated during the crisis as they would have done normally. The majority of farmers and firms of contractors received the compensation or payment amount that they were expecting after their animals were valued or work had been carried out. In the first four months, however, the outbreak placed huge strains on a small but significant number of the Department's systems of financial control. The Department has sought to correct overpayments and irregularities, although some disputes remain outstanding.

Figure 6 illustrates the many difficulties the Department experienced in paying farmers and procuring goods and services. Figure 7 sets out the steps the Department took to improve costs and financial control.

---

7   **The steps taken by the Department to improve cost and financial controls**

After the difficulties experienced in the early weeks of the crisis, **the Department took a number of actions to control the costs of procuring goods and services.** Specialist contract administrators and quantity surveyors were employed and dedicated teams were set up in Disease Control Centres to improve the cost effectiveness of operations. As a result, contract administration improved considerably and significant reductions in the rates paid for goods and services were achieved. The Department has also sought to recover value from surplus purchases.

During the crisis the **Department took steps to strengthen financial controls over payments.** A dedicated financial unit was set up to improve financial and accounting controls. Financial responsibilities were reorganised to relieve vets of involvement in financial matters and establish clearer lines of responsibility.

The Department has employed forensic accountants to examine the invoices of 107 of the largest contractors, including the 86 companies awarded contracts worth more than £1 million. In total these 107 companies have submitted invoices worth £474 million and to date the Department has paid £402 million in respect of these claims. The Department is withholding payment of the remainder until it is satisfied that contractors have provided sufficient evidence of work carried out.

By May 2002 the forensic accountants, quantity surveyors and contract managers employed are estimated to have saved the Department over £20 million. In addition, further savings have been generated through contract renegotiations and changes in invoicing practices as a result of work completed by the forensic accountants. A number of reductions have also been negotiated on accounts where investigation work is still in progress.

6 | The difficulties experienced in paying farmers and procuring goods and services

Problems with the slaughter compensation scheme increased the Department's costs. The Department has paid over £1.1 billion in compensation to farmers for the slaughter of their animals. Professional valuers determined the compensation to be paid. Their valuations tended to rise as more and more animals were slaughtered because they expected the resulting shortage of stock to be reflected in increased prices when the markets reopened. The Department's contingency plans envisaged the appointment of senior valuers to monitor valuations but no steps were taken to appoint such staff until July 2001.

The attempt to set standard rates for compensation contributed to a rise in prices. Standard rates for slaughtered animals were introduced on 22 March 2001 because the valuation process was thought to be delaying the slaughter of animals on infected premises. The Department expected that at least 70 per cent of farmers would accept the standard payment rates rather than seek individual valuations. In fact, however, the standard rates were used by only four per cent of farmers. Most chose to appoint a valuer. The standard rates acted as a floor for valuations and contributed to a rise in the compensation paid. The Department recognised that standard rates were not having the desired effect and withdrew them on 30 July 2001.

The Livestock Welfare Disposal Scheme helped many farmers but the generous rates created demand that exceeded initial capacity. The Department introduced the welfare scheme to alleviate the suffering of animals which were not directly affected by foot and mouth disease which could not be moved to alternative accommodation or pasture nor sent to market because of movement restrictions. Farmers received £205 million for the slaughter of two million animals. In setting up the scheme, the Department expected that farmers would pursue all other means of retaining or marketing their animals and turn to the scheme only as a last resort. This did not always happen, however. The rates were extremely attractive to farmers and the volume of applications overwhelmed the Rural Payments Agency, who administered the scheme. Demand for the scheme dropped off as movement restrictions were eased and financial incentives were reduced.

Many farmers and rural businesses suffered consequential losses. Farmers and rural businesses were not entitled to compensation for consequential losses. Farmers whose animals did not have foot and mouth disease, or were not deemed to have been exposed to the disease, or were not suffering from poor welfare conditions were not entitled to any payment. Many suffered greater financial hardship than farmers who met the criteria for payment as they had no extra money coming in to provide for those animals that they had to retain on their farms. Many rural businesses were also badly affected by the outbreak. The Government introduced a series of measures to alleviate the financial difficulties of small businesses.

The procurement of services and supplies was costly. Several factors combined to raise the Department's expenditure on goods and services to a much higher level than would have been incurred under normal conditions. The Department recognised that it might have to pay a premium to get things done at maximum possible speed. Valuers, slaughterers and private vets, without whom the disease could not have been eradicated, all demanded and received higher fee rates. The crisis conditions quickly led to shortages of equipment and materials and it was also difficult to find firms to undertake various services.

Some controls over purchasing were initially weak. Many contracts, which would normally be put out to tender, were awarded without competition. Aspects of some contracts were initially agreed orally. Labour, materials and services were ordered by telephone, fax, or e-mail, without having to go through the Department's full procedures for authorisation and approval and the provision of supporting paperwork. When some contracts came to be written and formalised it was sometimes difficult for the parties involved to recall the detail of what had been agreed. This later gave rise to many disputes about payment for work done.

Some financial controls were put under severe strain. Information was often lacking to support the payment of bills. The Department was frequently unable to monitor the work being carried out by contractors, especially the slaughter and disposal of animals, and the cleansing and disinfection of farms. Up to date information on current expenditure was not available at some local Disease Control Centres. Partly for these reasons, the Comptroller and Auditor General qualified his audit opinion on the 2000-01 resource accounts of the Ministry of Agriculture, Fisheries and Food.

The scale of the activity and the enormous task involved opened financial systems to the risk of fraud and abuse. The Department issued guidance to staff requiring allegations of fraud to be assessed. Where there was any substance to the allegations, cases were passed via regional managers to the Department's Investigation Branch. The Investigation Branch examined 33 allegations of fraud or abuse connected with the foot and mouth disease outbreak. Three cases are being prosecuted; 16 cases are still under investigation and 14 cases have been closed, either because the allegations were found to be unproven after investigation, or because there was insufficient evidence to warrant a prosecution, or because there were satisfactory explanations for the events that occurred.

Recommendations

12 **In the light of our examination and the findings set out above, we make the following recommendations. Although these recommendations are addressed specifically at controlling foot and mouth disease, they are also applicable in large measure to the control of other animal diseases. The Department already has in hand or has planned actions in response to many of the issues we have identified.**

Contingency plans need to be substantially revised

1 Contingency plans should be based on an analysis of the risks associated with an outbreak of foot and mouth disease. They should incorporate a range of different assumptions about the nature, size and spread of an outbreak. Plans should have regard to the economic, financial and environmental impacts of different methods of disease control.

2 A clear chain of command is required for handling any future crisis. Responsibilities, reporting lines and accountabilities need to be clearly defined in contingency plans, both at headquarters and locally.

3 The plans should include arrangements for the deployment of staff and the emergency purchasing of supplies and services. The Department should have access to key supplies and services and approved firms of contractors. Where possible, pre-agreed rates should be negotiated.

4 The Department should consult widely with central and local government, farmers and other major stakeholders about its contingency plans. The plans should identify the roles and responsibilities that each of these would have in the event of an emergency and how and at what point each would become involved.

5 Contingency plans should be tested on a regular basis at national and local level. Simulation exercises should involve appropriate stakeholders including local authorities, environmental agencies and farmers' representatives. The plans should be regularly reviewed and updated to ensure that they remain relevant in the light of any significant changes in the farming industry or elsewhere.

6 Communications and information systems need to be reviewed to ensure that they would be able to cope in an emergency.

In the event of a crisis, cost and financial control should not fall below a minimum standard

7 Clear procedures should be established for the procurement of supplies or services that are needed at very short notice. These procedures should include the arrangements for tendering, agreeing contracts and providing documentation.

8 In an emergency, key financial controls must remain in place to ensure that monies are properly accounted for, that the risks of fraud and abuse are minimised and that value for money is secured. There should be a clear audit trail with sufficient supporting documentation at all key stages.

Further research is required

9 Compensation and other payment schemes to farmers should be reviewed and revised as necessary to ensure that they operate fairly and provide value for money for the taxpayer.

10 Research should be undertaken into:

- The advantages and disadvantages of implementing a precautionary standstill of all livestock movements, the circumstances in which such a standstill should be implemented, and the timing of its implementation.

- The efficacy of biosecurity measures, including the need for footpath closures.

- The effectiveness and efficiency of the measures adopted to eradicate the disease and their appropriateness to local circumstances. This should include vaccination, methods of identification and diagnosis, culling policy, slaughter targets, and disposal methods for slaughtered animals.

11 In the light of the results of this research, the Department should review current animal health legislation to ensure that it meets current and likely future requirements for dealing with an outbreak of foot and mouth disease.

Follow-up action is required in a number of areas

12 The Department should urgently pursue those cases where it believes it was overcharged for goods and services. Irregularities in contractors' claims should also be investigated and resolved quickly.

13 Allegations of fraud or abuse during the crisis should be investigated thoroughly and any lessons learned incorporated into current guidance and procedures.

14 Disposal sites should continue to be subject to close environmental monitoring and inspection. The results should be published and reflected in the Department's contingency plans.

13 **There are also wider lessons for future contingency planning for all departments from the 2001 foot and mouth crisis. Departments need to be aware of the major threats in their areas of business and to manage those threats by having contingency plans in place which conform with best practice on risk management. Some key points for such contingency plans are set out in Figure 8.**

8   Key points on contingency plans for all departments

1 **Contingency plans need to be risk-based.** Plans should be informed by the identification of key risks and an analysis of the probability of their occurrence and what impact they might have. Planned responses should also be risk-based to ensure that proposed actions are proportionate and cost-effective.

2 **A range of different possibilities should be considered.** Plans should not be restricted to just the most likely scenario. The probability of other scenarios occurring, including a worst case, should also be assessed. Plans and proposed actions need to be flexible to enable an effective response to be made to unexpected scenarios.

3 **Stakeholders should be consulted.** Draft contingency plans should be discussed with key stakeholders from inside and outside government to ensure that all important aspects are covered and to secure broad agreement to the measures that would need to be taken. The draft plans should be shown to the Cabinet Office's Civil Contingencies Secretariat so that risks and combinations of risks that affect more than one Government department can be assessed. Once agreed, plans should be made readily available to stakeholders.

4 **A clear command structure should be prepared.** Plans should outline the command structure that would need to be introduced in a crisis. There should be clear lines of responsibility, reporting and accountability and structures to support logistics, liaison with other departments and stakeholders, and assessment of emerging risks.

5 **Access to key resources should be identified.** Plans should identify how personnel, goods and services of appropriate quality would be procured quickly and cost-effectively in the event of a crisis. Where appropriate, there should be reciprocal arrangements to draw in emergency personnel from other parts of Government and call-off contracts for essential supplies.

6 **Emergency cost and financial controls should be in place.** Plans should identify the basic controls that would need to be in place in a crisis so as to keep a tight rein over costs and to minimise the risks of fraud and abuse. The head of finance should be included in the emergency management team. This would enable opportunities to be seized quickly and ensure that financial considerations become an integral part of decision-making.

7 **Communications and information systems should be tested.** Communications and information systems need to be able to cope in crisis conditions. Systems for getting instructions to those in the field and for keeping stakeholders, the public and the media informed need to be reviewed and tested. Arrangements also need to be put in place for the systematic collection, assessment and dissemination of essential information that is required from the field. Staff should be trained in how to make the best use of communication and information systems in an emergency.

8 **Contingency plans should be tested and reviewed regularly.** Testing is essential to ensure that the measures to be taken are practical and effective; that staff know what to do in the event of a real crisis; and that plans are relevant and remain up to date in the light of experience. Certain test exercises should be designed to test the resilience of the plan's assumptions. The aim of the tests should be to learn lessons and develop experience of operating in the 'battle rhythm' of an emergency situation.

9 **With the onset of a crisis, contingency plans need to be immediately re-assessed.** Circumstances rarely replicate planned-for scenarios. At the outset of a crisis, facts should be gathered quickly and the plan's assumptions reviewed against the available information. The Civil Contingencies Secretariat should be invited to participate in this assessment.

executive summary

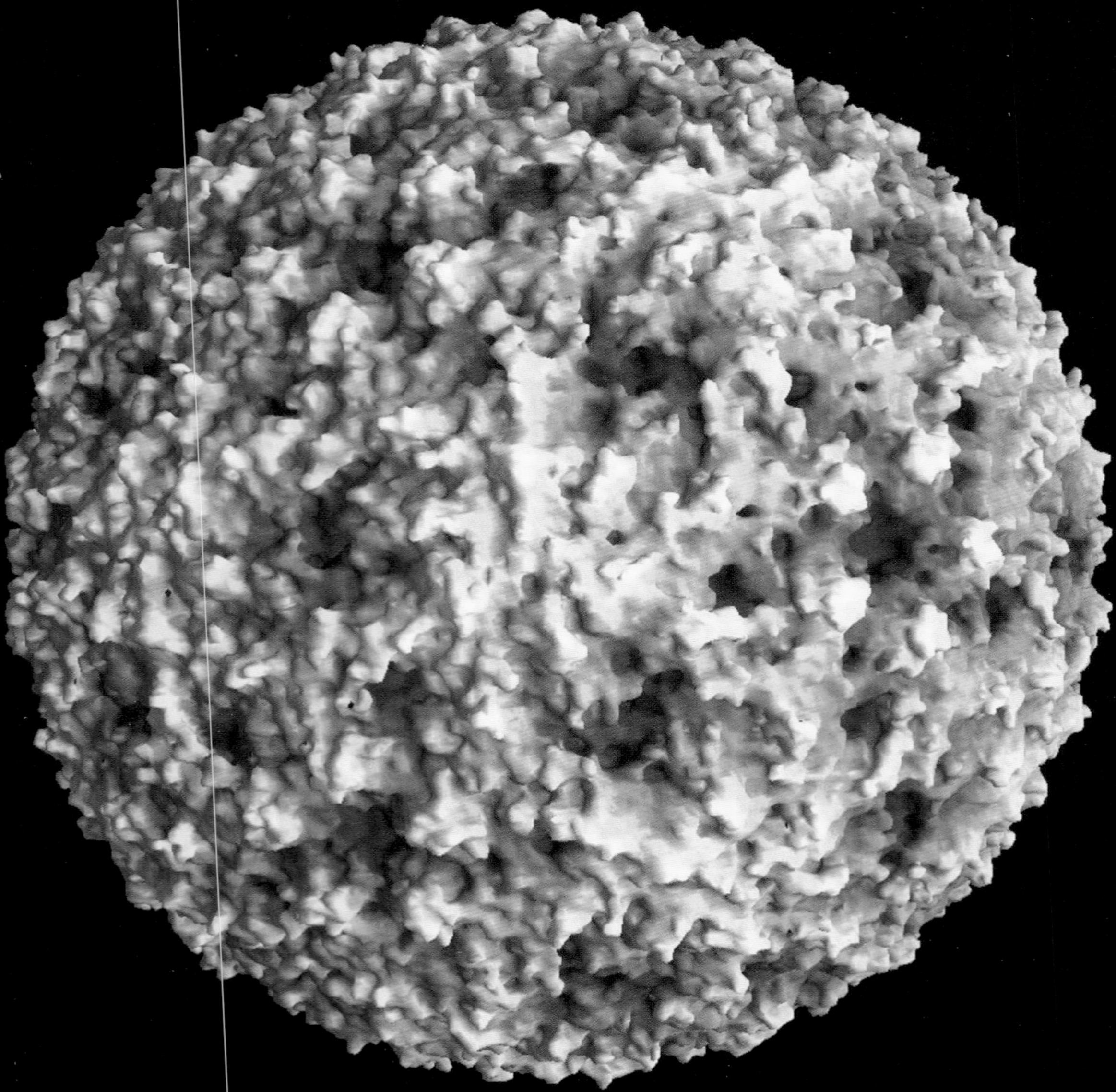

Part 1

Introduction

1.1 Foot and mouth disease was discovered in Britain in February 2001. Many agencies were involved in dealing with the outbreak, with the Department for Environment, Food and Rural Affairs (formerly the Ministry of Agriculture, Fisheries and Food) (the Department) taking the lead. Across the world there had never previously been an outbreak in sheep on the scale of the 2001 outbreak. As a result, the efforts involved in eradicating the disease were huge. From the early stages, the Prime Minister made it clear that combating the disease was the Government's top priority and whatever resources were needed should be obtained. Best value for money would be obtained by stamping out the disease quickly. The direct cost to the public sector is estimated at over £3 billion; and the cost to the private sector is estimated at over £5 billion. Against this background, we examined the adequacy of contingency planning for an outbreak of foot and mouth disease, how quickly and effectively the disease was eradicated and the cost-effectiveness of the action taken.

In the 2001 outbreak foot and mouth disease was widespread before the first case was suspected

The strain of virus that caused the 2001 outbreak of foot and mouth disease was highly infectious

1.2 Foot and mouth disease is a highly infectious viral disease that affects cattle, sheep, pigs, goats and other ruminants. Fever is followed by the development of blisters, mainly in the mouth or on the feet. Affected animals lose condition and may develop secondary bacterial infections. The most serious effects are seen in dairy cattle. The disease has a low mortality rate, except in young animals, though there are severe welfare implications both during and following infection. Though previously healthy animals may recover, they can be left with chronic infections, lameness, reproductive disorders and loss of milk yield. They may also continue to act as a source of infection.

1.3 Under favourable conditions the virus can survive for long periods. A very small quantity can infect an animal. Unchecked, the disease would quickly spread throughout a country between groups of animals in direct or indirect contact. Infected animals can excrete the virus for some days before clinical signs of the disease become evident and can remain infectious for a further week. The virus is present in fluid from blisters, and can also occur in saliva, exhaled air, milk, urine and dung. Animals pick up the virus by direct or indirect contact with an infected animal. Indirect contact includes eating infected products and contact with other animals, items or people contaminated with the virus, such as vehicles, equipment, fodder and anyone involved with livestock. Pigs, in particular, exhale large numbers of virus particles that can be transmitted in aerosol plumes.

1.4 The strain of virus responsible for the 2001 outbreak in Britain was the pan-Asiatic O type. This is highly virulent and has a short incubation period, with blisters appearing on infected animals within two to three days of infection. The clinical signs in sheep were highly variable in nature and often transient, making their detection difficult if a proper examination of sufficient animals was not carried out.

By the time the first case of the disease was suspected on 19 February 2001, the virus had already spread widely

Discovery and suspected source of infection

1.5 Suspicion of the disease was first reported on 19 February 2001 by an official veterinary surgeon after routine checks on pigs awaiting slaughter at the Cheale Meats abattoir, near Brentwood in Essex. The disease was confirmed at 8 pm on 20 February 2001, following a positive laboratory result. By 22 February 2001, the Department had undertaken some 600 tracings and had identified the likely source of the infection to a premises in Heddon-on-the-Wall in Northumberland, which had sent 35 sows to the Cheale Meats abattoir on 15 February.

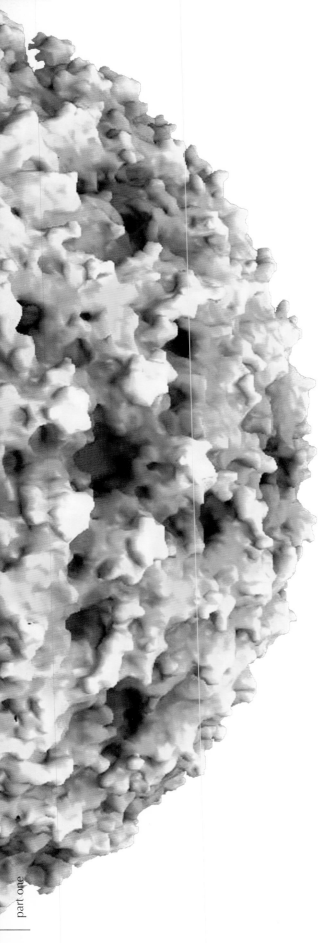

1.6 The Department's epidemiological investigations have since confirmed that the premises in Heddon-on-the-Wall was the most likely source case for the outbreak, because the signs of disease in pigs at this farm were the oldest on any infected premises in the outbreak. The most likely cause of transmission identified was the use of unprocessed pig swill. The Department has since banned the practice of feeding swill to pigs in the United Kingdom.

Seeding and geographical spread

1.7 Investigations by the Department established that the virus had spread from the farm in Northumberland to infect sheep on neighbouring farms. Sixteen sheep from one of these farms were sent to Hexham market on 13 February 2001 and then to other cattle markets **(Figure 9)**, including Longtown market near Carlisle (14-23 February) and Welshpool (19 February). The disease was spread further to Devon, Dumfries and Galloway, and Cheshire through livestock dealers and, subsequently, to markets at Hatherleigh (20 February), Hereford (21 February), Northampton (22 February) and Ross-on-Wye (23 February). At a time when the Department was unaware of the disease, infected sheep, and infective material on people, vehicles and equipment, had therefore been criss-crossing the country in hundreds of separate movements, putting them into contact with other livestock.

1.8 The Department's epidemiologists have now established that at least 48 premises in 15 counties had already been 'seeded' before 19 February 2001 when disease was first suspected. Disease had spread to a further nine premises and one county before confirmation on 20 February 2001. These were all the areas in which most cases of the disease subsequently occurred. Between confirmation and a national movement ban being imposed on 23 February 2001 another 62 premises are believed to have been infected, involving another seven counties. The main geographical spread of the disease had therefore occurred before any suspicion that disease may have been present in the country.

9 | **The spread of foot and mouth disease by livestock moved through markets before 23 February 2001**

Movement of foot and mouth disease infected animals before 23rd February 2001 and
location of implicated markets, abattoirs and dealers

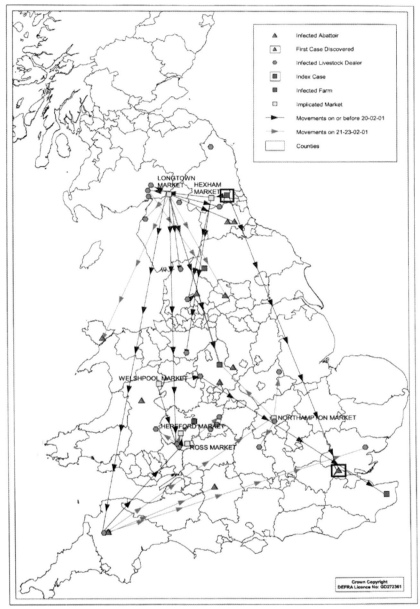

Subject to information available on 24/10/01

Source: Department for Environment, Food and Rural Affairs

Numbers of infected premises and animals slaughtered

1.9 The epidemic lasted for 32 weeks. The number of new outbreaks a day peaked at 50 on 30 March 2001. In late March 2001 **(Figure 10)** almost 300 cases were confirmed in a single week. Although the majority of areas were disease-free relatively quickly, the epidemic, overall, had a 'tail' caused by a series of separate discrete outbreaks. The last case was confirmed on 30 September 2001 on a farm near Appleby in Cumbria. On 14 January 2002, the Department announced that all counties were disease-free, though some individual farms remained under restrictions. On 22 January 2002, the international animal health organisation, the Office Internationale des Epizooties, re-instated the United Kingdom on the list of countries free of foot and mouth disease. On 5 February 2002, the European Commission lifted remaining meat and animal export restrictions; a partial relaxation of the ban on exports of pig, sheep and goat meat from certain parts of Britain had been made in autumn 2001. A chronology of events over the course of the outbreak is at Appendix 1.

1.10 Some 2,026 premises in Britain were officially declared infected (1,722 in England, 187 in Scotland and 117 in Wales). There were outbreaks in 44 counties, unitary authorities and metropolitan districts **(Figure 11)**. Worst

10 New confirmed cases[1] by week of the 2001 outbreak (Week 1 is 20-26 February)

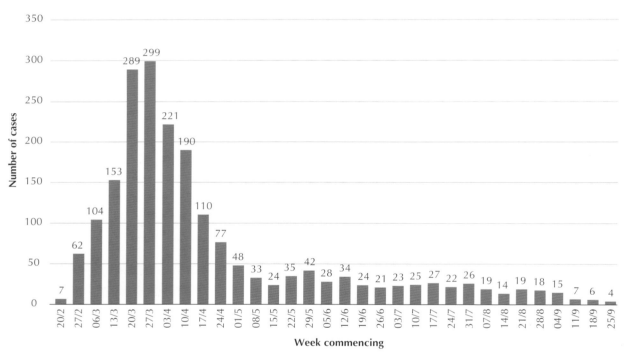

NOTE

1. Infected premises

Source: Department for Environment, Food and Rural Affairs

affected were Cumbria (with 893 infected premises), Dumfries and Galloway (176), Devon (173) and North Yorkshire (133). Animals were slaughtered on over 8,000 further premises where it was believed that livestock had been exposed to the disease.

1.11 More than 6 million animals were slaughtered over the course of the outbreak. Some 4.2 million animals were culled for disease control purposes and 2.3 million animals were culled and paid upon for welfare reasons[4] or under the light lambs scheme[5] (**Figure 12**). Farmers received compensation for animals slaughtered for disease control purposes and payments for animals culled for welfare reasons or under the light lambs scheme. The above figure of 6 million does not include many slaughtered new born lambs and calves, that were not counted in the Department's database because their value, for compensation purposes, was included in the valuation assigned to their mother. The Department told us that they have been unable to estimate the numbers of lambs and calves involved.

11 **The distribution of foot and mouth disease infected premises across England, Scotland and Wales during 2001**

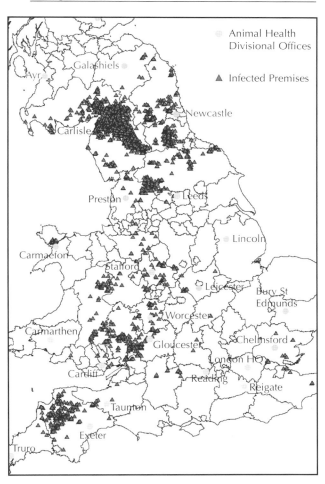

NOTE

Disease Control Centres were set up at Animal Health Divisional Offices in those divisions with infected premises. A new Disease Control Centre was also set up in Newcastle. In Dumfries and Galloway, the Disease Control Centre was based at the Animal Health Divisional Office at Ayr, but there was also an operational centre at Dumfries, close to the centre of the local outbreak.

Source: Department for Environment, Food and Rural Affairs

12 **Animals slaughtered for disease control and welfare purposes**

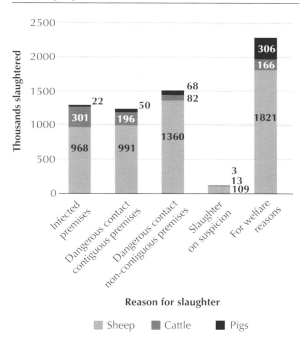

Reason for slaughter

■ Sheep ■ Cattle ■ Pigs

NOTES

1. The totals for dangerous contact non-contiguous premises include the three-kilometre cull.

2. The totals slaughtered for welfare reasons include 1,768,000 sheep, cattle and pigs under the Livestock Welfare (Disposal) Scheme and 525,000 lambs under the Light Lambs Scheme.

3. The figures exclude around 4,000 other animals, chiefly goats and deer, slaughtered for disease control purposes and around 3,000 other animals for the Livestock Welfare (Disposal) Scheme.

4. The figures exclude many slaughtered new born lambs and calves who were not counted in the Department's database because their value, for compensation purposes, was included in the valuation assigned to their mother.

Source: The Department for Environment, Food and Rural Affairs and the Rural Payments Agency.

4   On 22 March 2001 the Department introduced the Livestock Welfare (Disposal) Scheme. This voluntary scheme was intended to alleviate the suffering of animals who were not directly affected by foot and mouth disease but could not be sent to market because of movement restrictions.
5   From 3 September 2001 until 26 October 2001 the Rural Payments Agency operated a scheme to slaughter lambs which could not be marketed because of the ban on exports and other movement controls and which could otherwise have faced serious welfare problems.

part one

17

1.12 To set these figures into context, at the time of the agricultural census in June 2000 there were 40 million sheep, nine million cattle and six million pigs in Britain. In a normal year, around 18 million sheep, 13 million pigs and 2.5 million cattle would be slaughtered for food. In 2001, despite the difficulties caused by foot and mouth disease, there was still commercial slaughtering for the food chain of 13 million sheep, 11 million pigs and 2.2 million cattle.

Other parts of the European Union were affected by the 2001 outbreak

1.13 The 2001 outbreak of foot and mouth disease spread to France, the Republic of Ireland, the Netherlands and Northern Ireland (**Figure 13**). These places benefited from the knowledge that disease was near from daily reports made by the Department to the European Union on the developing situation in the United Kingdom. This forewarning enabled them to carry out intensified surveillance and controls over livestock markets, to increase border checks and to carry out precautionary slaughter of livestock that had originated recently from Britain based on information supplied by the Department. Their responses to outbreaks included the preventive culling of animals in "at risk" premises near infected premises. In the Netherlands, there was ring

vaccination around the whole cluster of infected premises; and the animals involved were subsequently slaughtered. This tactic was adopted partly because there was insufficient rendering and logistical capacity to carry out a preventive cull within a four-day target.

The scale and impact of the 2001 epidemic was greater than that of the last serious outbreak in Britain in 1967-68

1.14 The last serious outbreak of foot and mouth disease in Britain was in 1967-68[6]. It lasted seven months and involved 2,364 infected premises and the slaughter of 442,000 animals. There were significant differences between the two outbreaks, however: the 2001 outbreak was a national epidemic initially disseminated by sheep, whereas the 1967-68 outbreak mainly affected cattle in the dairy farms of the Cheshire plain. The features of the 1967-68 epidemic and comparisons with 2001 are set out in Appendix 2. Foot and mouth disease was eradicated in the European Union in the late 1980s, which permitted an end to vaccination in continental Europe in 1991. Since 1991 there have been outbreaks in the European Union in 1993, 1995, 1996 and 2000. Foot and mouth disease is endemic in parts of Africa, Asia, the Middle East and South America.

13 **Outbreaks of foot and mouth disease in the European Union in 2001**

Country	Number of infected premises	Animals slaughtered	Number of animals slaughtered per infected premises	Duration of outbreak (first and last confirmed cases)
France[1]	2	58,000	29,000	12 to 23 March 2001
Republic of Ireland[1]	1	60,000	60,000	22 March 2001
The Netherlands[1]	26	268,000	10,300	21 March to 22 April 2001
Northern Ireland	4	50,000	12,500	1 March to 22 April 2001
Great Britain[2]	2,026	4,200,000	2,070	20 February to 30 September 2001

NOTES

1. France, Ireland and the Netherlands were re-instated on the Office Internationale des Epizooties' list of countries free of foot and mouth disease on 19 September 2001.

2. The figure for animals slaughtered in Great Britain excludes 2.3 million animals slaughtered for welfare reasons or under the light lambs scheme.

Source: National Audit Office.

6   *There was an outbreak of the disease in 1981 in the Isle of Wight, on a cattle farm. The source of infection was windborne transmission from Britanny, in northern France. Aware of a potential risk, the Department had instigated heightened vigilance, including advice and publicity to the industry. As a result of this advice, there was prompt reporting of the case by the farmer and the immediate action by the Department restricted this outbreak to one premises.*

Many agencies were involved in dealing with the 2001 outbreak

There is an international and legal framework for dealing with animal health

1.15 Control of animal disease is undertaken within the context of guidance produced by two intergovernmental bodies, the Office Internationale des Epizooties and the European Commission for the Control of Foot-and-Mouth Disease. The first, with 158 member countries, sets sanitary rules for international trade in animals and animal products and disseminates veterinary scientific information on animal disease control. The second, established under the auspices of the Food and Agriculture Organisation of the United Nations, promotes research and co-ordination of national control programmes among 33 European member countries.

1.16 There are two aspects to the legal framework for controlling foot and mouth disease: European Union **(Figure 14)** and domestic legislation. The Animal Health Act 1981 and the Foot and Mouth Disease Order 1983 (as amended) (SI 1983/1950) were in force at the time of the 2001 outbreak. The Act states that the Minister may cause to be slaughtered any animals affected with foot and mouth disease or suspected of being affected or any other animals that appear to have been exposed to the infection, and requires farmers of slaughtered animals to be paid compensation. The Order sets out rules to be observed at infected places and in areas subject to disease control restrictions (infected areas and controlled areas).

14 **The European Union framework for control of foot and mouth disease**

European Community law sets out in Council Directives the framework within which Member States of the European Union deal with foot and mouth disease. Commission Decisions cover detailed measures and are made with the advice of national veterinary experts meeting in the European Union's Standing Veterinary Committee.

Council Directive 85/511/EEC of 18 November 1985, amended by 90/423/EEC of 26 June 1990, requires Member States to respond to an outbreak of foot and mouth disease by means of restrictions on movement of livestock, agricultural produce, people and vehicles, other biosecurity[7] measures and slaughter of animals at the agricultural holding concerned in order to 'stamp out' the disease. In some cases, emergency vaccination can also take place. Council Directive 90/423 requires Member States to draw up contingency plans for dealing with foot and mouth disease.

Source: National Audit Office

The Ministry of Agriculture (the Department) took the lead in dealing with the outbreak

1.17 At the time of the outbreak, the Ministry of Agriculture, Fisheries and Food (the Department) was the central authority for animal health matters in England and Wales. Since June 2001 these functions have been the responsibility of the Department for Environment, Food and Rural Affairs. At the time of the outbreak, the organisational structure of the Department as regards animal health matters was as set out in **Figure 15 overleaf**. It comprised an animal health policy-making wing and an operational wing, the State Veterinary Service. Many other parts of the Department were also involved from the beginning of the outbreak.

1.18 Under the Scotland Act of 1998, legislation on all animal health matters has been devolved to the Scottish Parliament and policy development and implementation made the responsibility of Scottish Ministers. During the 2001 outbreak, Scottish Ministers operated within an agreed policy framework whilst taking account of local circumstances.

1.19 The position in Wales is more complex. Some, but not all, animal health functions were transferred to the National Assembly for Wales in 1999, but the operational 'on the ground' disease control functions in the Animal Health Act 1981 and the Foot and Mouth Disease Order 1983 continued as functions of the Department post-devolution. These functions included such matters as slaughter, seizure of carcasses and the declaration of infected areas. Under the Animal Health Act 1981, the National Assembly for Wales makes secondary legislation jointly with the Department and makes regulations under section 2(2) of the European Communities Act 1972, mainly to implement Community decisions on import and export of animal carcasses and animal products. During the 2001 outbreak decisions affecting Wales were in practice taken by the Department in consultation with the National Assembly.

1.20 Under concordats with the Scottish Executive and the National Assembly for Wales, the State Veterinary Service provides the national veterinary service for the whole of Britain. Its operational responsibilities include notifiable disease control, the import and export of animals and animal products, farm animal welfare and public health safety on farms. It was led by the Chief Veterinary Officer; and the service delivered through local Animal Health Divisional Offices, headed by Divisional Veterinary Managers. The range of duties includes liaising with farmers, local authorities, private veterinary surgeons, market operators, transporters,

---

7   In the context of the foot and mouth disease outbreak, biosecurity refers to the precautions taken to minimise the risk that the virus might be spread inadvertently by those working with livestock and visiting farms, and after infected animals have been slaughtered and disposed of. This includes thorough cleansing and disinfecting of the person, equipment and vehicles by those working on and visiting farms, minimising inessential contact with susceptible animals and cleansing and disinfecting of premises that have been infected.

slaughterhouses and the general public. Field service staff deal with outbreaks of notifiable disease, carry out welfare visits to farms and markets and advise farmers on disease prevention.

The Prime Minister oversaw the development of policy

1.21 From the outset, the Prime Minister was closely engaged, receiving regular briefings on the developing situation and the control strategy, and holding meetings with Ministers and stakeholders. Once the national scale of the outbreak was clear, the Prime Minister, with the Cabinet and the Minister of Agriculture, oversaw the development of policy. On 12 March 2001 the Prime Minister made it clear that combating the disease was the Government's priority and whatever resources were needed should be obtained. Best value for money would be obtained by stamping the disease out quickly. On 22 March 2001, the Cabinet Office Briefing Room was set up to oversee disease strategy and operations.

15 **The Department's organisational structure (animal health) on the eve of the 2001 outbreak**

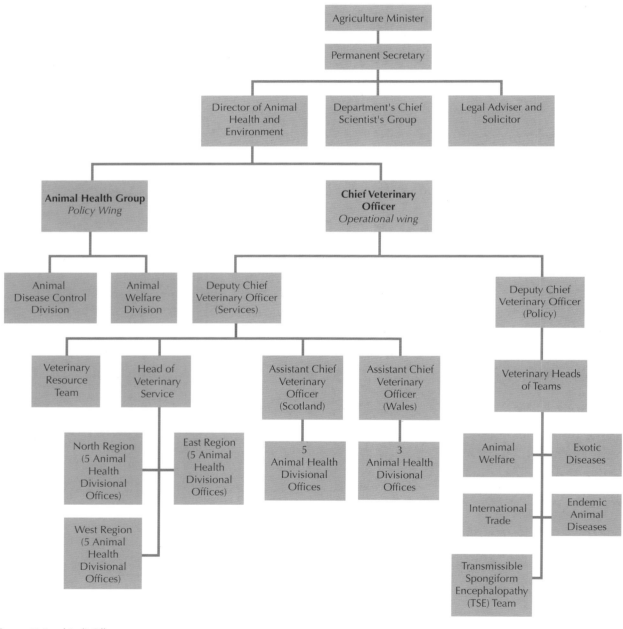

Source: National Audit Office

Many other departments and agencies were also involved

1.22 The huge scale and impact of the 2001 epidemic meant that many other organisations became involved in helping the Department in its fight to contain and eradicate the disease. Agencies of the Department, other government departments and agencies, non-departmental public bodies and local government bodies were closely involved. Private contractors and voluntary and stakeholder groups - for example, the Royal Society for the Prevention of Cruelty to Animals and the National Farmers' Union - also played important roles. Some of the public sector and related bodies involved are set out in **Figure 16**. Many of these bodies were also represented within the Department's Joint Co-ordination Centre. Other departments and agencies also assisted, for example, by providing advice and loaning staff.

The scale of the 2001 outbreak was enormous and the costs were huge

The cost to the public sector is estimated at over £3 billion

1.23 The Department has calculated that the direct cost to the public sector of eradicating the 2001 outbreak of foot and mouth disease was over £3 billion (**Figure 17**). This figure is equivalent to around 0.8 per cent of annual public expenditure. The costs have been funded from the government's contingency reserve.

1.24 Up to 60 per cent of the United Kingdom's spend on disease eradication activities, including compensation to farmers, may be recouped from the European Union's budget[8]. However, if the records supporting the claims are not sufficiently robust the European Commission may conclude that some of the expenditure is not eligible and therefore reduce the amount of reimbursement. In June 2001, the United Kingdom submitted an initial claim based on estimated costs of £1,153 million. An updated reimbursement claim for £998 million, based on costs of £1,663 million, was submitted in October 2001. £735 million of the claim is for compensation payments to farmers for animals slaughtered and for destruction of contaminated feeding stuffs. The other £263 million of the claim is for cleansing and disinfecting of farms and for transport and haulage and disposal of livestock. On 28 February 2002, the Department received an advance payment of £217 million from the Commission; in the meantime, European Union auditors continue their work on the first part of the claim for compensation paid to farmers.

---

8   *In practice, the rules relating to the special budget rebate obtained during the 1980s (known as the 'Fontainebleau abatement'), mean that Britain funds 71 per cent of any money given. Consequently, the net amount that can be recouped is effectively 17 per cent (60 per cent of 29 per cent).*

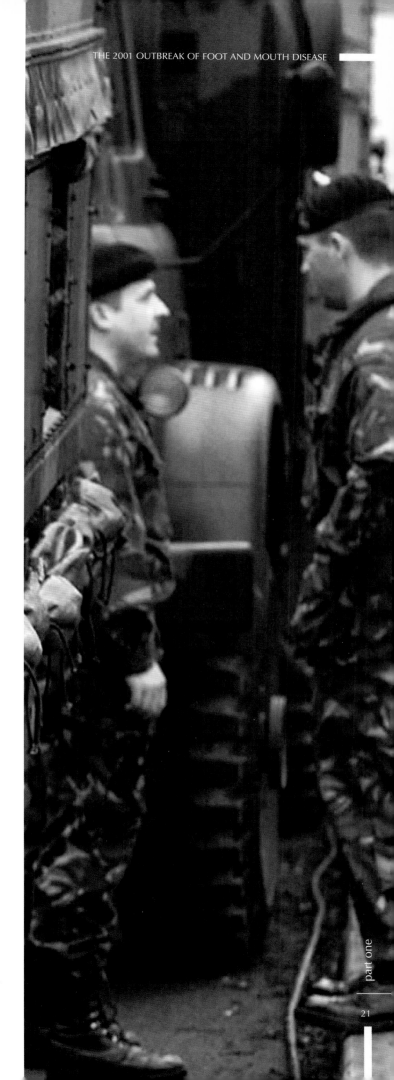

16   **Some of the main public sector bodies that assisted the Department during the 2001 epidemic**

Name	Role in the outbreak
Other government departments	
Cabinet Office	From the beginning, responsible for sorting out actions that involved more than one department. From 22 March 2001, serviced the Cabinet Office Briefing Room. The Cabinet Office's News Co-ordination Centre acted as a central information source, with its own website. Government Offices for the Regions: Their staff were seconded to Disease Control Centres, providing important administrative manpower support, including for external communications. They liaised on tourism and rural economy issues. [Before 7 June 2001, the Government Offices for the Regions were co-ordinated by the Department of Environment, Transport and the Regions].
Department for Culture, Media and Sport	Liaised with and supported the tourism sector, providing around £18 million to the British Tourist Authority and English Tourism Council for research and promotional work.
Department of Environment, Transport and the Regions (in June 2001 parts became the Department for Transport, Local Government and the Regions and other parts merged with the Ministry of Agriculture, Fisheries and Food to form the Department for Environment, Food and Rural Affairs)	Contributed to development of carcass transport arrangements and advised on planning, air and environment quality issues relating to disposal of carcasses and clean up. Supported the Rural Task Force, which was set up on 14 March 2001 to advise the Government on the impact of foot and mouth disease on the wider rural economy. The Rural Task Force comprised representatives from a range of Government departments and agencies and from stakeholder bodies, such as tourism, farming, small business, local government, community interests and conservation. It was chaired by the Environment Minister until June 2001 and by the Rural Affairs Minister thereafter.
Department of Health	Working with other agencies, including the Public Health Laboratory Service, the Centre for Applied Microbiology and Research, the Environment Agency and the Food Standards Agency, assessed risks to human health posed by disease control activities, such as slaughter and disposal of animals; provided information and advice to health professionals and the public; investigated suspect human cases of foot and mouth; monitored risks and produced surveillance reports; and assisted the Department with laboratory testing.
Department of Trade and Industry	Scientific advice provided by the Government's Chief Scientific Adviser, Head of the Office of Science and Technology. The department-sponsored Regional Development Agencies and Small Business Service were closely involved in help provided to non-farming businesses via a Business Recovery Fund.
Ministry of Defence	From mid-March 2001 the armed services assisted, centrally and locally, in organisation and logistical arrangements, particularly in slaughter, transport and disposal. Around 2,000 troops were deployed to Disease Control Centres in late April and early May.
The devolved administrations	
National Assembly for Wales	Contributed to policy decisions in London. From 26 March 2001 provided a regional operations director and operations directorate, including administrative and information technology resources. Administered movement licensing schemes. Provided helplines, websites, advice and support to affected sectors.
Scottish Executive	Responsible for disease control in Scotland and contributed to policy decisions in London. From 20 March 2001, provided a regional operations director, set up on 26 March a disease strategy group (comprising vets, administrators and the armed services), and provided administrative and technical resources. Administered own movement licensing schemes. Provided helplines, websites, advice and support to affected sectors.
Local government bodies	
Local Authorities	Responsible for enforcement of the Animal Health Act and Orders. Local authority animal health and trading standards officers monitored and enforced compliance with the Animal Health Act. Determined when to close and re-open rights of way and erected restriction notices and signs. Issued certain movement licenses. Provided information through websites and assistance to local businesses.

Name	Role in the outbreak
Police	Up to 1,000 officers were involved in general outbreak-related policing duties at various times, such as ensuring public order during protests at mass burial sites. Participated, alongside local authority trading standards officers and the Department's staff, in intensified biosecurity patrols within Yorkshire and Cumbria.
Agencies, non-departmental public bodies and other government-supported bodies	
Environment Agency (A non-departmental public body) Scottish Environment Protection Agency	Gave environmental advice to assist decisions about the disposal of carcasses and other waste. This included advice on safe locations for burial to minimise the risk of groundwater pollution and on the use and disposal of disinfectants.
Food Standards Agency	Gave advice on food safety issues, including the potential implications of pyre disposal sites. Conducted monitoring for dioxins in food around such sites. Its Executive Agency, the Meat Hygiene Service, introduced and supervised the 'Direct to Slaughter Scheme' on behalf of the Department for animals sent to red meat slaughterhouses for human consumption. The Scheme required the Meat Hygiene Service to approve abattoirs to operate under the Scheme; undertake additional ante and post mortem inspection; ensure that all animals were killed within 24 hours of arrival and that none were returned to farms; and supervise the cleansing and disinfection of livestock vehicles.
Institute for Animal Health (funded by a core grant from the Biotechnology and Biological Sciences Research Council and from contracts, including with the Department)	The Institute's Pirbright Laboratory is a United Nations Food and Agriculture Organisation-designated and an Office Internationale des Epizooties-designated World Reference Laboratory for foot and mouth disease. It is the only United Kingdom facility licensed by the Department to hold and work with live foot and mouth disease virus. The Institute is responsible for global surveillance of foot and mouth disease and hosts the International Vaccine Bank for foot and mouth disease. During the 2001 epidemic, the Institute's Pirbright Laboratory tested diagnostic samples sent in by the Department's vets from animals suspected of having the disease. It also carried out tests for serological surveillance. The Institute also provided expert advice, formulated and tested the emergency vaccine and worked with the Met Office to predict airborne spread of the virus.
Meat and Livestock Commission (A non-departmental public body)	Licensed and supervised the operation of cleansing and disinfecting centres for the Long Distance Movement Scheme. Organised transport and supervised abattoirs for the Livestock Welfare (Disposal) Scheme. Administered licensing schemes for sheep shearers, scanners and dippers. At the peak of the outbreak, provided 450 staff to the Department at commercial rates.
Met Office (a Trading Fund of the Ministry of Defence)	Provided advice from the outset on airborne disease risk to inform the Department's epidemiological modelling, and advice on smoke from pyres and detailed site-specific weather forecasts.
Rural Payments Agency (formerly the Intervention Board to 16 October 2001) (Executive Agency of the Department)	Administered the Livestock Welfare (Disposal) Scheme and Light Lambs Scheme. Played a major part in organising the disposal of carcasses.
Veterinary Laboratories Agency (Executive Agency of the Department)	Provided vets and scientific advisers and developed veterinary risk assessments. Co-ordinated the introduction of sero-surveillance and provided information technology links and software to all serology providers. Carried out serological surveillance testing at its Penrith, Luddington and Shrewsbury laboratories, as well as loaning staff to the Institute for Animal Health at Pirbright. Provided procurement and stores supply services to the Department's Animal Health Offices and Disease Control Centres throughout the country, including sampling equipment, protective clothing, firearms and ammunition.

Source: National Audit Office

1.25 Other public bodies incurred costs additional to those shown in Figure 17. These include:

- losses of normal income - for example, from local authority-owned tourism attractions and, in the case of the Meat and Livestock Commission, a 22 per cent fall (to £25 million) in slaughter levy income collected in 2001-02;

- loss of tax revenues;

- grants (amounting to over £100 million) to assist with training, business advice and recovery for affected businesses; and deferred tax and business rates (£242 million); and

- the potential costs of cancelled or delayed work, such as cattle tuberculosis testing and flood defence maintenance.

The cost to the private sector is estimated at over £5 billion

1.26 In March 2002 the Department estimated that the epidemic cost the private sector over £5 billion[9]. At the height of the outbreak, in March to April 2001, a quarter of all businesses reported some adverse impact from the crisis. However, many of the losses suffered by individuals and firms gave rise to equivalent amounts being spent elsewhere in the economy. Consequently, the net economic impact of the outbreak was less. The Treasury estimated in November 2001 that the net economic effect was less than 0.2 per cent of gross domestic product (this would be equivalent to less than £2 billion). Factors that would have specifically impacted on gross domestic product are a reduced number of foreign tourists, holidays taken abroad rather than in the United Kingdom, the loss of some meat and livestock exports, and increased meat imports.

17 **Direct costs to the public sector of the 2001 outbreak of foot and mouth disease**

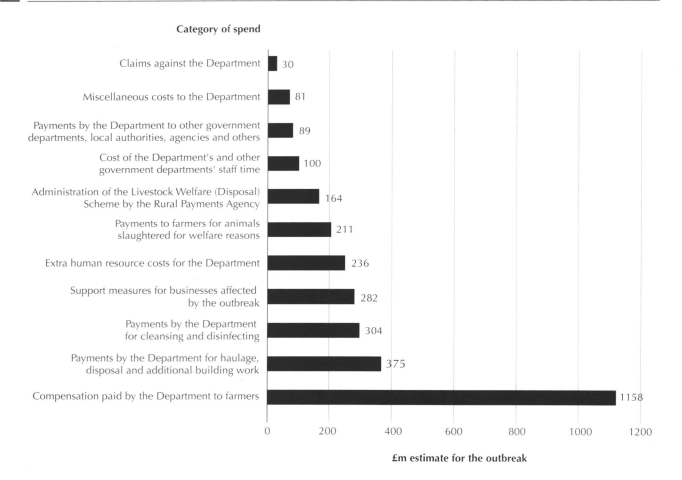

Category of spend

Category	£m
Claims against the Department	30
Miscellaneous costs to the Department	81
Payments by the Department to other government departments, local authorities, agencies and others	89
Cost of the Department's and other government departments' staff time	100
Administration of the Livestock Welfare (Disposal) Scheme by the Rural Payments Agency	164
Payments to farmers for animals slaughtered for welfare reasons	211
Extra human resource costs for the Department	236
Support measures for businesses affected by the outbreak	282
Payments by the Department for cleansing and disinfecting	304
Payments by the Department for haulage, disposal and additional building work	375
Compensation paid by the Department to farmers	1158

£m estimate for the outbreak

Source: The Department's forecast as at 24 May 2002 of the likely overall costs of dealing with the 2001 outbreak of foot and mouth disease.

9   *The Economic Cost of Foot and Mouth Disease in the United Kingdom: a joint working paper (the Department and the Department for Culture, Media and Sport, March 2002).*

1.27 After taking account of compensation and other payments to farmers, the Department has estimated that the outbreak cost agriculture and the food chain over £600 million. This figure is made up of £355 million in respect of agricultural producers - equivalent to a fifth of their annual income; £170 million in respect of the food industry - auction markets, abattoirs, processors and hauliers; and £85 million representing the indirect impact on the agricultural supply sector. The National Farmers' Union has separately estimated the uncompensated losses to the agricultural sector at £900 million.

1.28 Tourism suffered the largest financial impact from the outbreak, estimated by the Department and the Department for Culture, Media and Sport to have been between £4.5 and £5.4 billion. Businesses directly affected by tourist and leisure expenditure are estimated to have lost between £2.7 and £3.2 billion; and there was a further impact of between £1.8 and £2.2 billion on industries and services that are supported by tourism.

1.29 One element of the loss, the net effect of which is estimated at over £400 million, resulted from a drop in foreign visitors (**Figure 18**). Between March and May 2001 there was a fall of around 15 per cent in holiday visits to Britain by overseas residents. Thirty per cent of domestic visitors also changed their travel plans as a direct result of the outbreak. Rural Cumbria, Devon and Northumbria were hit worst, but the overall impact masks significant variations both between localities and between different businesses. Some domestic tourist expenditure was redirected to market towns and coastal resorts, and abroad. Precautionary closure of many rights of way meant that rural bed and breakfast enterprises were particularly hard hit.

The outbreak had the potential for serious damage to the environment and implications for human health

1.30 As a result of the precautions taken and the responses made to potential and actual problems arising, the Environment Agency and the Department of Health judge that the impact of the outbreak on the environment and human health appears to have been short-term and localised, although monitoring is continuing. There were over 200 water pollution incidents reported in England and Wales, although only four were major and none are expected to have long-term impacts. In Scotland there were no reported water pollution incidents related to the outbreak. Monitoring of mass burial sites indicated that there were no major health problems caused by pollution of private or public water supplies. There were also no reported human gastro-intestinal problems linked to the outbreak.

Comprehensive monitoring of the air quality around the six major pyres found no evidence of failures to meet national air quality standards.

1.31 The Department has been concerned, however, about mental health problems that may have been caused by the outbreak and has awarded £250,000 to North Cumbria Health Authority to carry out research into the human cost of the disease. In March 2002 the Scottish Executive announced £50,000 in funding for the Royal Scottish Agricultural Benevolent Institution to assist with local counselling services.

18 **Fall in spending by overseas visitors during the peak months of the 2001 foot and mouth outbreak compared with the same months in 2000**

Up to a half of the fall in spending shown may have been attributable to the foot and mouth disease outbreak

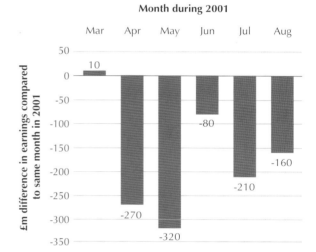

NOTES

1. Figures are seasonally adjusted to take account of holidays, such as Easter, falling at different times of the year.

2. Treasury analysis suggests that up to a half of the fall in overseas visitor numbers during 2001 was attributable to the outbreak of foot and mouth disease.

3. Figures for later months are not shown as a result of the distorting impact on international travel of the 11 September 2001 terrorist attacks in New York and Washington.

Source: Overseas Travel and Tourism, First Release (Office for National Statistics, 10 May 2002).

We examined how the 2001 outbreak of foot and mouth disease was handled

Issues, scope and methodology

1.32 Our investigation into the handling of the outbreak addressed three broad questions:

■ How well prepared was the Department to deal with an outbreak on the scale that occurred?

■ How quickly and effectively was the disease eradicated?

■ Recognising the difficult conditions under which the Department was operating, was action taken in a cost-effective manner and were there adequate controls against irregularity?

1.33 We did not examine:

■ the source of the outbreak - this is the subject of a continuing investigation by the Department;

■ the controls needed to prevent infectious animal diseases from being imported into the United Kingdom - this is partly the subject of a scientific review by the Royal Society (see below); and

■ the recovery process - it is too soon to assess the efforts made by the Government and others to assist the farming industry in its recovery from the disease.

1.34 The investigation covered England, Scotland and Wales, since the Department took the lead in controlling the outbreaks in these parts of the United Kingdom. It did not cover Northern Ireland, which has its own animal health legislation and veterinary service. We carried out the fieldwork for the investigation in late 2001 and early 2002 at a time when Departmental officials and many of the other individuals and organisations we questioned were fully stretched dealing with the direct impact and aftermath of the outbreak. We are most grateful to those who provided us with information in such difficult circumstances. Our methodology is set out in full in Appendix 3.

There have been a number of other inquiries into the 2001 outbreak

1.35 On 9 August 2001 the Government announced three independent inquiries:

■ An **Inquiry into the lessons to be learned from the foot and mouth disease outbreak of 2001** and the way the Government should handle any future major animal disease outbreak. The inquiry is being chaired by Dr Iain Anderson and is due to report in July 2002.

■ An **Inquiry by the Royal Society into Infectious Diseases in Livestock**, to review scientific questions relating to the transmission, prevention and control of epidemic outbreaks of infectious disease in livestock. The review is being chaired by Sir Brian Follett and is due to report in July 2002.

■ A **Policy Commission on the Future of Farming and Food,** to advise on how to create a sustainable, competitive and diverse farming and food sector. The commission was chaired by Sir Don Curry and reported in January 2002.

The terms of reference and working methods of these inquiries are described in Appendix 4.

1.36 There have also been:

■ Completed local public inquiries organised by Devon and Northumberland County Councils and investigations by Gloucestershire and Shropshire County Councils. A local public inquiry announced in February 2002 by Cumbria County Council is due to report at the end of July 2002.

■ Hearings and a report by the House of Commons' Environment, Food and Rural Affairs Committee.

■ An inquiry, by the Royal Society of Edinburgh, into the outbreak in Scotland, the control procedures employed and the impact on the Scottish economy. The inquiry is due to report in July 2002.

■ A report by the National Assembly's Agriculture and Rural Development Committee on the handling of the foot and mouth epidemic in Wales.

■ Reports on aspects of the outbreak by a range of government and stakeholder bodies, including the Environment Agency, the Countryside Agency, English Nature, the Farm Animal Welfare Council and the National Farmers' Union of England and Wales.

1.37 In February 2002, the European Parliament established a cross-party 'Temporary Committee' on the 2001 outbreak of foot and mouth disease. It will assess European Union policy on foot and mouth disease control, the handling of the epidemic in the United Kingdom and other European Union countries and the cost to the European Union budget. It will also consider the controls necessary on meat imports from third countries.

1.38 Additional information on the 2001 outbreaks in Scotland and Wales is at Appendices 5 and 6. The performance results of local Disease Control Centres are set out in Appendix 7.

Part 2

Preparing for a possible outbreak of foot and mouth disease

2.1 Thorough and effective contingency planning is crucially important for the control of foot and mouth disease. Essential tactical and strategic decisions still need to be taken during an outbreak in response to how that outbreak is developing. Nevertheless, the more effective the preparations, the more effective that response is likely to be.

2.2 This Part of the Report examines the Department's preparations for a possible foot and mouth epidemic. We found that:

- the nature and scale of the 2001 outbreak were unprecedented (paragraphs 2.3 to 2.6);

- the Department had prepared contingency plans for foot and mouth disease which met European Union requirements (paragraphs 2.7 to 2.13);

- the Department's contingency plans were not sufficient to deal with an outbreak on this scale (paragraphs 2.14 to 2.61); and

- following eradication of the disease, the Department is revising its contingency plans (paragraphs 2.62 to 2.64).

The nature and scale of the 2001 outbreak were unprecedented

2.3 The nature, scale and impact of the epidemic of foot and mouth disease that hit Britain in 2001 were unprecedented. The United Kingdom authorities faced a monumental task in eradicating the disease. It is unrealistic to expect that any contingency plan could have coped with all the problems and difficulties that occurred. The Department believes that in the circumstances no country in the world could have been prepared for an outbreak on this scale and that no amount of contingency planning could have fully prepared the Department for the events that unfolded. Certainly, the epidemic went well beyond the planning assumptions of international veterinary agencies.

Other countries would have faced similar difficulties

2.4 All countries with livestock carry out contingency planning for foot and mouth disease. The Australian Chief Veterinary Officer has said that the nature and magnitude of the foot and mouth events in Britain were such that any country would have struggled under the circumstances. Countries such as Australia, Canada, New Zealand and the United States, and other Member States of the European Union are revising their contingency plans as a result of the experiences of their staff during the outbreak in Britain.

2.5 In response to questions from the European Parliament's Temporary Committee on the 2001 outbreak of foot and mouth disease, the European Commission has stated that, "Contingency plans are drawn up on the base of a risk assessment. There is no Member State that bases the contingency plan on more than 2,000 outbreaks with about 50 new outbreaks per day for several weeks. The whole calculation made for the European Union estimated in a worst case scenario 13 primary outbreaks, each with about 150 secondary outbreaks, throughout the Community over 10 years. Experts also estimated that the likelihood of virus introduction into the United Kingdom would be extremely low. It cannot be reasonably expected from any Member State to design a contingency plan for the event of an epidemic causing more outbreaks within months than the 10 years estimate for the whole of the Community."

2.6 Mr David Byrne, the European Commissioner for Health and Consumer Protection, told the Committee on 25 March 2002:

> "The reality is that from the very first moments the authorities, especially in the United Kingdom, faced a monumental task in eradicating the outbreak.
>
> All Member States were required to have a contingency plan in place to deal with potential outbreaks of foot and mouth disease. These plans were reviewed and approved by the Commission. Nonetheless, nobody envisaged an epidemic on a scale of over 2,000 outbreaks. This was considered unthinkable, especially on an island Member State considered especially well positioned to keep out the virus.
>
> I have also noted more than once that perhaps the pre-occupation with BSE (Bovine Spongiform Encephalopathy) over-stretched veterinary services. Certainly, any proposal to strengthen measures in relation to foot and mouth disease before the last year's outbreak would have been considered a diversion from the political priority attached to BSE."

The Department had prepared contingency plans for foot and mouth disease

2.7 Since before 1967 the Department has had field instructions for veterinary and other staff on the practical measures to be taken in the event of an outbreak of foot and mouth disease. These instructions had been used since before 1967, being updated as necessary.

The Department's contingency plans met European Union requirements

2.8 The European Commission requires Member States to draw up a plan specifying the national measures to be implemented in the event of an outbreak of foot and mouth disease (Article 5 of Directive 90/423). In 1991 the Commission set out criteria to be applied in drawing up the plan and provided guidance on how the criteria could be met (**Figure 19**). The Commission approved a Member State's plan if it was satisfied that the criteria had been met. It is up to each Member State to decide what further measures may be needed in proportion to identified risks.

19   **European Commission requirements for contingency plans for foot and mouth disease**

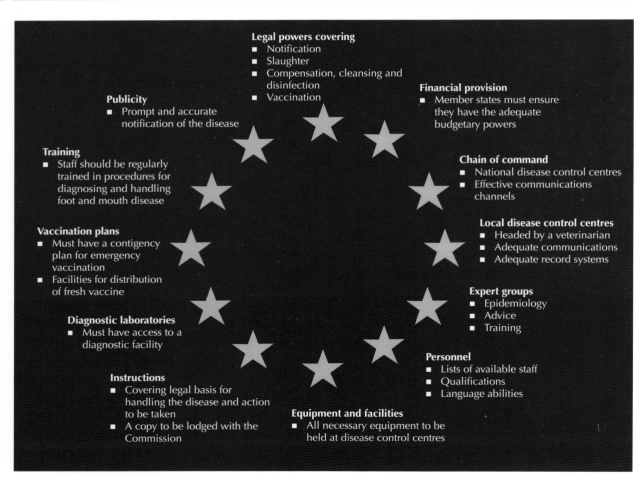

2.9 In 1992 the Department submitted to the European Union its contingency plans for Great Britain. The plans comprised a national contingency plan, local contingency plans prepared by Animal Health Divisional Offices, and standing field instructions. The plans were approved by the Commission on 23 July 1993. Contact names and telephone numbers and minor facts were updated in July 2000. The contingency plan describes how the authorities in Britain would deal with an outbreak of foot and mouth disease, and in particular:

■ the legal powers and financial provisions within which the Department would operate;

■ the chain of command and the relative powers of a National Disease Control Centre (the Department's headquarters) and local Disease Control Centres; and

■ the arrangements for personnel resources, staff training, diagnostic laboratories, publicity and disease awareness.

The emphasis of the Department's contingency plans was on local action to deal with outbreaks of the disease

2.10 The main responsibility for local contingency planning falls on Animal Health Divisional Offices. Much therefore depends on local initiative and thoroughness. We found that each Animal Health Divisional Office had prepared a local contingency plan that mirrored the national plan on a local scale. Local plans provided useful information in the event of an emergency, such as the location of large livestock units, the actions to be taken if disease is found in a market and firms of suppliers that could provide goods and services. The plans also set out the roles of staff in Animal Health Divisional Offices and the names and telephone numbers of local contacts, for example, the Environment Agency, local authorities and police. Local staff were required to ensure that the contingency plans were kept up to date. At the time of the February 2001 outbreak, 19 divisional plans had been updated within the previous year, although four - those for Chelmsford (January 1999), Leicester (1999-2000), Lincoln (1997-98) and Reading (July 1996) - had not.

2.11 The Department's standing instructions for veterinary and other field staff (Veterinary Instructions, Procedures and Emergency Routines) provide guidance on dealing with diseases and other tasks performed by the veterinary service. "Chapter 3" details the arrangements for dealing with suspected and confirmed cases of foot and mouth disease. The arrangements cover: testing; imposing movement restrictions; tracing the spread of the disease; valuation; compensation and slaughter; disposing of carcasses; cleansing and disinfecting of infected premises; and establishing and staffing disease control centres. They are continually updated as

required. An electronic version of "Chapter 3" was available on the Department's intranet from February 1999 for vets and other members of staff to consult. During the 2001 outbreak, "Chapter 3" was supplemented by over 300 Emergency Instructions to reflect knowledge and experience gained in combating the disease in the field. The Emergency Instructions provided guidance on the implementation of policy as it developed during the outbreak. They covered issues such as diagnosis, epidemiology, culling policies, animal welfare, licensing of animal movements and cleansing and disinfecting.

Contingency plans worked in areas where there were relatively few cases

2.12 Contingency plans were put into operation during the 2001 epidemic and worked for many of the outbreaks around the country. The outbreaks were eliminated rapidly in some counties, such as Essex, Kent, Leicestershire, Northamptonshire, Oxfordshire and Warwickshire. In these counties there were few infected premises - only 26 in total - and there was little or no spread of the disease.

2.13 In some of the worst hit areas of the country, however, especially Cumbria, Devon and the North East of England, the Department's contingency plans proved inadequate for the circumstances. The unprecedented scale of the outbreaks in these areas meant that the resources needed to deal with the disease rapidly went beyond what had been envisaged in the contingency plans.

The Department's contingency plans were not sufficient to deal with an outbreak on this scale

The Department had assessed the main risks of an exotic disease such as foot and mouth entering the country but had not undertaken a specific risk assessment of foot and mouth disease

2.14 Good risk management requires the identification of key risks, an assessment of the probability of their occurrence and likely impact, and consideration of what preventive or contingency measures, if any, are proportionate and appropriate. In September 2000 the Department produced a report on procedures for risk analysis, which recommended that arrangements for risk analysis should:

■ identify that coverage of risk is comprehensive;

■ ensure that policy making in the light of the risk identified is sufficiently rigorous and innovative; and

■ ensure that the risks identified are periodically examined and appropriate action taken.

2.15 The Department had applied good practice on risk management to many areas of its work. But because of other priorities and a shortage of available resources, it had not undertaken a specific risk assessment on foot and mouth disease. However, the Animal Health Group within the Department had assessed the main generic risks of an exotic disease, such as foot and mouth, entering the country. This included the risks to human health and animal welfare, and the economic and financial risks.

2.16 There are essentially three areas of risk to be considered in the prevention of an outbreak of exotic disease: disease entering the country; susceptible animals accessing infection; and disease spreading within the country. The Department considers that these had been addressed by risk assessments, appropriate risk management procedures and legislation for:

■ import controls on animals and animal products;

■ controls on swill premises and vehicles;

■ controls on animal movements;

■ identification of animals during movement and recording such movements; and

■ cleansing and disinfecting of livestock vehicles and markets.

2.17 With finite resources, there has to be a correlation between the level of risk of an event and the priority that can be given to addressing that risk. National and international advice and opinion was that the risk of an initial incursion of foot and mouth disease into the United Kingdom was low. The Department believed that its existing generic risk assessments and risk management would act to address the threat of animal disease entering the country and subsequently becoming established and spreading.

Over time the Department has sought to address changing features of modern farming practices

2.18 Some aspects of farming practices have changed considerably since 1967-68:

■ The volumes of cattle and particularly sheep movements had increased dramatically in recent years and increased the possibility that, if undisclosed infection was present in the country, there could be widespread dissemination of cases. By the time the 2001 outbreak was discovered, it had already spread far and wide.

■ There had been specialisation, contraction and increased veterinary supervision of the slaughtering industry. An example of this specialisation was the abattoir in Essex where the disease was first detected in 2001. It had, for many years, taken cull sows from all over the United Kingdom as it was able to comply with export requirements and handle the animals involved.

2.19 The Department has introduced legislation including on animal movements, identification and traceability, hygiene and veterinary standards in the slaughterhouse industry, cleansing and disinfection, and the detection and notification of animal diseases. The legal and environmental framework for disposal of animal by-products including carcasses had changed significantly since 1967-68. The Department's plans recognised the need for disposal of carcasses to take place in ways acceptable to the Environment Agency and local authorities. The working assumption was that on-farm burial and, failing that, on-farm burning were the preferred methods of disposal as these present the lowest risk of disease spread. Later, the rendering of carcasses became the preferred route.

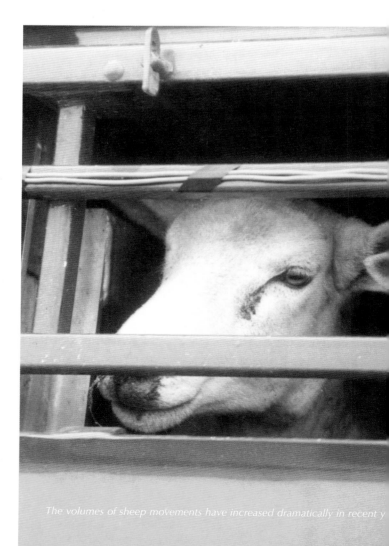

The volumes of sheep movements have increased dramatically in recent y...

The implications of vaccination could have been more fully considered in contingency plans

2.20 European Union policy towards foot and mouth disease has been that outbreaks of the disease should be stamped out by slaughter. Routine vaccination of livestock to prevent or slow the course of foot and mouth disease is not legal in the European Union. However, European Union law permits the use of emergency vaccination, with European Commission authorisation, as part of a stamping out policy when foot and mouth disease has been confirmed, threatens to become extensive, and where vaccination would be an appropriate measure to help eradicate the disease. The European Commission requires Member States to establish facilities that will allow the prompt distribution and administration of vaccine and requires that contingency plans should give details of vaccine requirements in the event of an emergency.

2.21 The Department considers that emergency vaccination of cattle is inefficient as a means of controlling foot and mouth disease on its own, because the time taken after innoculation before immunity develops allows significant spread of the disease from infected premises, and thus requires a wide vaccination ring to be drawn.

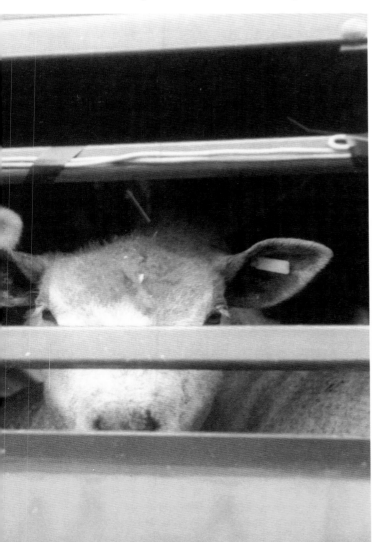

Moreover, vaccination alone cannot eradicate the virus. The Department believes that emergency vaccination may not always be an appropriate tool for controlling outbreaks in other species.

2.22 During the 2001 outbreak the European Commission gave the Netherlands permission to use emergency suppressive ring vaccination in conjunction with the later slaughter of the animals. Vaccination helped the Netherlands to stem the 2001 outbreak. It also allowed the disposal of carcasses to be managed effectively because vaccinated animals could be slaughtered as and when facilities were available. The outbreak in the Netherlands was, of course, on a very much smaller scale than in Britain and the area of infection easier to identify. Because the vaccination ring was necessarily drawn widely, the methods used in the Netherlands resulted in the slaughter of more animals per infected farm than in Britain: about 10,000 animals per infected farm compared with 2,000 per farm in Britain. The Department considers that any similar vaccinate-to-kill policy in Britain would have been less cost-effective than the slaughter policy adopted because it would have resulted in more animals being slaughtered with associated costs and disposal implications. Because of the extent of the spread of the disease the Department believes that ring vaccination would not have been effective in controlling the 2001 outbreak.

2.23 The Department's contingency plan for Britain noted that the International Vaccine Bank, set up in 1985 at Pirbright, would be equipped to deal with emergency vaccine supplies. The plan stated that Britain would vaccinate up to 500,000 cattle in the event of an emergency vaccination. However, details of the strain of vaccine and numbers of doses required cannot be predicted before an outbreak. A set of Instructions ("Chapter 3A") covering action to be taken if vaccination were to be used had been prepared in 1998, but these were not issued to vets in local offices. This meant that the information could not be used as a basis for local planning and preparedness, although any vaccination programme would have to be co-ordinated and resourced nationally.

2.24 In mid-March 2001, when the 2001 outbreak was at its height, the Government accepted that there might be a case for a limited emergency vaccination programme and the Department began to draw up plans to vaccinate cattle in Cumbria and Dumfries and Galloway and possibly Devon. The programme was intended to protect cattle, including those that were due to move out from winter sheds, as the risk of their becoming exposed to infection from contaminated pastures or other livestock would be increased. It was a 'vaccinate to live' plan, with the cattle not to be prematurely slaughtered. The Department obtained permission from the European Union's Standing Veterinary Committee to apply emergency vaccination. Operational plans for carrying out the vaccination were drawn up by ADAS Consulting Limited and potential teams put on stand-by. In Scotland the Scottish Agricultural College was commissioned to put potential vaccination teams on standby.

2.25 In preparing the vaccination plans efforts were made to address the concerns of farmers, consumers, retailers and food manufacturers. The use of vaccination was controversial for several reasons, including:

■ The success of a vaccination policy was open to doubt. The Government's Chief Scientific Adviser proposed a limited cattle vaccination plan for cattle over-wintering in sheds in Cumbria in mid-April 2001, subject to certain conditions which in the event could not be met. The proposal was supported by the Chief Veterinary Officer. The Chief Scientific Adviser advised the Prime Minister that broader vaccination of sheep would be unlikely to be successful. There were no internationally recognised and validated tests able to distinguish between vaccinated and infected animals and it would therefore be difficult to tell how far the virus was present in the country's livestock. The Department estimated that the 500,000 doses of vaccine drawn from the International Vaccine Bank would be sufficient to complete the vaccination of cattle in the heavily infected areas of north Cumbria and Devon. But it would not be enough for a nationwide campaign in all other infected areas.

■ There are major practical implications in carrying out vaccination. Considerable resources would be required, which may put pressure on veterinary and technical staff carrying out disease diagnosis and eradication. There would need to be active co-operation by stock owners for the identification, gathering, handling and vaccination of animals.

■ Vaccinated animals would have to be under restrictions for movement and certain breeding procedures. Compliance with the restrictions would require industry co-operation and further resources to monitor, police and enforce. Before any products from a vaccinated animal could enter the food chain it would require further processing. All milk would have to be pasteurised and meat would need to be deboned and matured.

■ Many farmers were concerned that vaccination would, for a defined period, prevent Britain from being able to export meat and livestock to key markets. Farmers' unions were opposed to vaccination because of the possible impact on domestic and export markets and the conflicting scientific opinion on the issue.

■ Consumers might be reluctant to buy meat or milk from vaccinated animals. The Food Standards Agency considered that there were no risks to human health from the consumption of meat or milk from vaccinated animals. However, concerns were raised by the food industry about the effect of vaccination on trade, particularly in the export market.

2.26 The Department took steps to provide information on vaccination: its website contained the information and scientific advice provided to the Prime Minister; a booklet on the subject was sent to all livestock farmers in England; and the issue was raised at local and national stakeholder meetings. On 26 April 2001 the Department announced that it would not vaccinate without the support of a substantial majority of the farming community, veterinarians, the wider food industry and consumers. The National Farmers' Union expressed serious reservations about the Cumbria vaccination plan and by the end of April 2001, with the number of new confirmed cases falling steeply, the Department considered that the need for immediate vaccination had passed. The use of vaccination continued to remain an option to deal with local hotspots during later stages of the epidemic if considered appropriate, and plans and resources to implement them remained in place.

2.27 The Department spent time at the height of the outbreak trying to get stakeholder support for a programme of emergency vaccination. The Department would have been in a better position if the issues surrounding emergency vaccination had been considered in the Department's contingency planning and clear strategies prepared and agreed on the circumstances in which it might be used. Such an assessment would have included an analysis of the costs and benefits of vaccination alongside the available alternatives, such as culling. The Department believes that it would have been extremely complicated, if not impossible, to produce a strategy for all species and eventualities.

2.28 In the Netherlands, contingency plans for dealing with an outbreak of foot and mouth disease were drawn up following an outbreak of classical swine fever in 1997. These included contingency plans for vaccination and the trigger points at which vaccination would be used. Even so, detailed contingency plans for emergency vaccination were only prepared after the outbreak of foot and mouth disease in Britain and before the disease was confirmed in the Netherlands.

2.29 The future role of vaccination is being considered at the European Union level. The United Kingdom will contribute to discussions on a new Directive to control foot and mouth disease which is likely to be issued by the European Commission later in 2002. The Commission is expected to take account of the experience of the 2001 outbreak and to recognise that the response to future outbreaks has to be rapid and flexible and might include emergency vaccination.

The plans were based on the most likely scenario and other scenarios were not considered

Scale of the epidemic

2.30 The Department's contingency plans complied with European Commission minimum specifications. This requires that each Member State should ensure that it has immediately available sufficient trained staff to deal with up to ten infected premises at any one time and to maintain proper surveillance in protection zones three kilometres in radius around each. The Department considered two scenarios in its planning carried out in 1993, both involving ten infected premises: a moderate scenario, which suggested a requirement for 232 field vets; and a severe scenario involving greater numbers of livestock and requiring 347 field vets. After this review, the staffing level for vets was set at around 230 field vets, where it remained through to 2001.

2.31 The Department felt that this was a sensible basis for planning because the nature of outbreaks in Europe during the 1990s suggested that most outbreaks would involve only a small number of infected premises at the outset. In 1967-68 there were 24 separate primary outbreaks, although between 1991 and 2001 there were on average only 2.1 outbreaks each year in Europe. There was awareness of a growing world-wide threat from the pan-Asiatic O strain of foot and mouth disease and an increased risk of its introduction to disease free countries. The virulence of the disease was made apparent in 1997, when Taiwan suffered a very large outbreak, involving the infection of four million pigs, nearly 40 per cent of the country's entire pig population. However, information provided by the Office Internationale des Epizooties in 2000 indicated that, although there was a risk that the strain would reach Western Europe via the Middle East and Turkey, it would give rise to only a few cases. In addition the European Commission for the Control of Foot-and-Mouth Disease, under the auspices of the United Nations Food and Agriculture Organisation, considered that the risk of foot and mouth disease being introduced to the United Kingdom was low.

2.32 The Department told us that, if there had been up to 10 infected premises in 2001, the contingency plans would have worked. In the event, however, there were at least 57 infected premises before the initial diagnosis was made and over 2,000 infected premises in total. The Department considers that no amount of scenario planning would have envisaged the sequence of unprecedented and improbable events that led to an outbreak on the scale of that in 2001.

2.33 The European Commission's requirements on preparing contingency plans represent one scenario of preparedness. They do not preclude Member States from taking further action to prepare for disease outbreaks and to devise different methods and approaches according to the severity, incidence and nature of particular outbreaks and in proportion to the risks that such outbreaks might occur. We found that the Department had not considered a range of different scenarios. Although scenario planning might not have envisaged an epidemic on the scale of that in 2001, it would nevertheless have alerted the Department to the dangers that it faced if the number of outbreaks turned out to be significantly greater than the ten allowed for in its contingency plans.

Nature of the epidemic

2.34 **Figure 20 overleaf** lists some of the factors that contributed to the 2001 outbreak being of the scale and nature that it was. The outbreak was characterised by a series of unusual and highly unlikely events. The probability of any of these individual events occurring was low but their impact, particularly when they occurred together, was catastrophic. It would not be possible or proportionate to counter all such factors. Nevertheless, it is important that the consequences of such factors are addressed in future contingency planning. Such consideration would place the Department in a better position to respond to an outbreak.

The impact of a large-scale outbreak on non-farming businesses was not addressed in contingency plans

2.35 Because the Department's contingency plans did not consider other, worse, scenarios than ten cases at a time, little prior consideration was given to the wider effects that a large scale epidemic might have. At the beginning of the 2001 outbreak, the potential impact on tourism was not fully appreciated. The combined effect of public perceptions and media reporting of the outbreak and the initial blanket closure of most footpaths by local authorities **(see Figure 21 on page 35)** and the time taken to reopen them, had a very severe effect on the rural tourist industry in some areas. The potential impact on other countryside users and non-farming businesses of a large-scale outbreak of foot and mouth disease and the appropriate response was not considered as part of wider Government contingency planning. Nevertheless, the impact on tourism was recognised early in the outbreak, with the Countryside Agency issuing a first estimate of the impact on rural businesses on 1 March 2001. The Department for Culture, Media and Sport issued guidance on visiting the countryside for tourism, sport or recreation on 5 March 2001. On 6 March 2001 Ministers of key departments met at the Tourism Summit to review the impact of foot and mouth disease. On 13 March 2001 the Prime Minister chaired a meeting on the impact of foot and mouth disease on the rural economy attended by Ministers and representatives of organisations representing rural tourism, such as the British Tourist Authority, the National Trust and the Youth Hostels Association.

20   Characteristics of the 2001 outbreak

Characteristic	Consequence	Action by the Department (both before and during the 2001 outbreak)
Initial outbreak of disease not reported quickly.	The disease was not reported on the farm where the outbreak is believed to have originated. Disease was seeded around the country.	It was an offence not to report suspicion of a notifiable disease.
Disease would be in a species in which the strain of virus did not always cause obvious clinical signs.	Unlike the 1967-68 outbreak, which mainly involved cattle, the 2001 epidemic was predominantly in sheep in which clinical signs were sometimes difficult to detect.	Advice was provided to farmers and vets very early in the outbreak advising of clinical signs and the difficulty of identifying them in sheep.
An outbreak occurring at a time of high animal movements.	The outbreak occurred at a time of the year when high numbers of sheep were being moved through markets.	Long distance movements of animals occur throughout the year and the movement of only one infected animal is sufficient to spread disease. Interim movement arrangements introduced in the autumn of 2001 now impose a standstill period between journeys, thereby allowing more time for any disease to be noticed.
Tracing of legitimate livestock movements difficult and illegal movements impossible.	Sheep movements were harder to trace than cattle or pig movements.	For all species there is a requirement for movements to be recorded.
Shortage of vets for identifying infected animals.	The scale of the epidemic resulted in the Department soon running out of vets.	Action was taken to overcome the shortage but it took time to select, recruit and train suitable staff.
The time taken to obtain test results on suspected infected animals.	Where slaughter was carried out only after laboratory confirmation of a clinical diagnosis, delays in receipt of results would delay slaughter.	From 21 February 2001 where it was possible the Department would confirm cases of infection on clinical grounds rather than waiting for laboratory test results.
Some people would ignore biosecurity measures.	A minority of farmers and others did not comply with biosecurity requirements leading to local and long distance spread of the disease.	Later creation of Restricted Infected Areas raised awareness of biosecurity by strict policing and enforcement of existing legislation. In spite of this, breaches of biosecurity still occurred.
Infected animals not slaughtered quickly enough.	In the early stages there were logistical and resource limitations which delayed slaughter in some cases.	Full compliance with the restrictions in place on premises where animals were awaiting slaughter would greatly have reduced the risk of spread of the disease.
On-farm burial and burning of carcasses not practicable.	To minimise the risk of disease spread the preferred method of disposal was on-farm burial and burning. This proved impracticable because of environmental constraints and the high water table in some areas.	The Department quickly carried out risk assessments and introduced biosecurity protocols so as to be able to use alternative routes of disposal.

Source: National Audit Office and Department for Environment, Food and Rural Affairs

21 **Footpath closure**

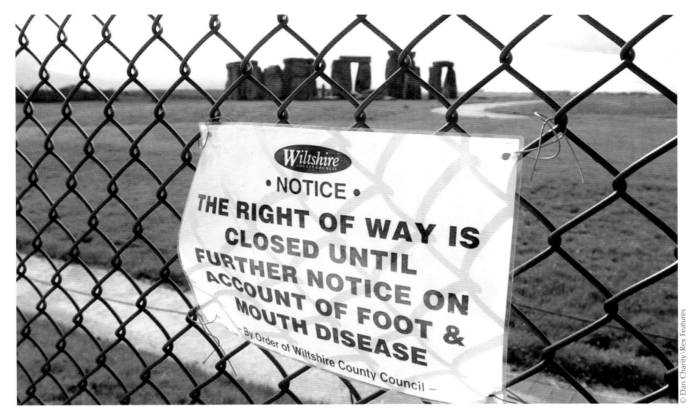

© Dan Charity/Rex Features

The 240,000 kilometres of public rights of way in Britain are significant in attracting visitors to rural areas. At the start of the 2001 outbreak, with the potential scale of the epidemic unknown, the Government advised the public to stay off farmland and avoid contact with farm animals. On 27 February 2001 local authorities were empowered by Statutory Instrument to close footpaths and bridleways where necessary not only in infected areas but also outside them, subject to clearance with the Department.

Almost all local authorities adopted a precautionary approach and used the powers given to carry out blanket closures of all paths without having to erect signs on individual paths. By early March 2001 almost all footpaths were closed, including some in towns, woodland and across arable land. Counties such as Buckinghamshire, Lincolnshire and East Sussex which were disease-free were among those that kept their footpaths closed for the longest periods.

The impact on rural tourism was huge, although this was not due solely to footpath closures. In some areas visitor numbers fell to nothing. The most severe impacts were probably on small accommodation providers, such as bed and breakfast establishments, guesthouses and owners of self-catering accommodation. Walking, climbing and mountaineering were severely curtailed. The Youth Hostels Association told us that they estimated a consequent net loss of income of about £5 million, as occupancy levels of their rural hostels fell by 35 per cent on the preceding year. The Youth Hostels Association decided that, in order to make good the losses suffered as a result of foot and mouth disease, and to safeguard its capacity to invest for the future, 10 Youth Hostels would be closed and sold.

The Rural Task Force examined the impact of the outbreak on tourism, including how far the damage to countryside tourism was caused by foot and mouth disease and how much by other reasons. The Rural Task Force found that although it was difficult to apportion the downturn in visitor numbers between foot and mouth disease and other factors, the loss of domestic visitors to the countryside was exacerbated by the poor spring weather, but arose in the first place

mainly because of the almost complete closure of footpaths, suspension of sports such as fishing, cancellation of rural events, and closure of many country houses and other visitor attractions. The impact lasted longer than necessary owing to the slowness of some local authorities in reopening footpaths. The perception that the countryside was closed continued long after it had ceased to be the reality. The fall in overseas visitors may have reflected the high pound and economic slowdown in the USA and Japan, but was above all because of the images of the disposal of carcasses, particularly the "mega-pyres" shown in the foreign media.

From late March 2001, the Government encouraged local authorities to reopen footpaths in areas free from disease while asking walkers to adhere to good practice guidelines on their safe use. In Scotland, the Scottish Executive distributed a "Comeback Code". This followed a veterinary risk assessment which concluded that the risk of disease transmission by walkers was extremely small. However, progress with reopening was slow. By Easter, on 15 April 2001, only 14 per cent of the network was open and by 17 May 2001 around 26 per cent of footpaths were open. In late April 2001, the Countryside Agency was provided with £3.8 million to assist local authorities and National Parks with reopening costs.

On 23 May 2001, local authorities were issued with guidance to reopen most rights of way outside the three kilometre protection zones around infected premises. By 25 June 2001, two-thirds of footpaths were open and on 20 July 2001, after consulting local authorities, the Government revoked remaining blanket closures. By February 2002 99 per cent of footpaths had been reopened.

The Department's new interim contingency plan for dealing with foot and mouth disease in the future envisages that the countryside would be kept "open". The blanket approach to footpath closures would not be repeated. Footpath closures would only be authorised in particular circumstances based on specific veterinary risk assessments.

Recommendations from previous animal health reports had largely been adopted with the exception of some recommendations from an internal report in 1999

Northumberland report on the 1967-68 outbreak of foot and mouth disease

"Our main recommendations and suggestions relate to the need for more detailed pre-outbreak planning for the mobilisation of manpower and equipment to deal with an outbreak wherever it may occur. The plans should provide for the swift and effective mobilisation of manpower and resources,... and for smooth expansion to deal with outbreaks no matter what dimensions they assume." (Northumberland Report, Part 2, paragraph 218)

2.36 In 1969 the Duke of Northumberland reported on the Department's handling of the 1967-68 epidemic of foot and mouth disease. Part One of his report set out seven recommendations and Part Two a further 105 recommendations for dealing with future outbreaks. The recommendations covered areas such as veterinary practice, administrative arrangements, slaughter, disposal, compensation and communications. The Department's contingency plans largely reflected the recommendations set out in the Northumberland report, some of which were subsequently endorsed in European Union and United Kingdom law.

2.37 We have examined four instances where it did not appear that the Department had fully followed the Northumberland report's recommendations. The Department told us that, 30 years on from the report, its plans for dealing with an outbreak had been modified to

some degree compared to the 1969 report's recommendations. For example, the Northumberland report recommended that:

■ *"Contingency plans for the application of ring vaccination should be kept in constant readiness. They could be put into operation should our recommendations in II [for changes in the conditions of meat import policy] not be successful in limiting the number of outbreaks (Part 1, Recommendation IV)."* The Department considers that the situation had changed radically since Northumberland's day. The changes in meat import conditions had contributed to a significant reduction in the number of foot and mouth outbreaks since 1968. The disease had also effectively been eradicated at European Union level. This led the European Union to prohibit the use of vaccination against foot and mouth disease by Member States except in an emergency, subject to Commission Decision. The Department had prepared field instructions on the action to be taken if vaccination were to be used. The Department told us that these had not been issued to field staff along with the rest of the foot and mouth disease instructions because of the need to obtain prior European Union authorisation for any vaccination campaign. The Department considers nonetheless that the Northumberland report's recommendation was in substance met by the outline arrangements in place.

■ *"A comprehensive plan should be in readiness for the mobilisation of resources within and outside the Department in the event of an outbreak of foot and mouth disease. One of the main objectives of the plan should be to relieve veterinary officers of non-veterinary work (Part 2, Recommendation 5)."* As envisaged by the Northumberland report, arrangements had been put in place to relieve veterinary staff of the control of labour and machinery engaged on disposal and cleansing and disinfection, although at the outset of the outbreak veterinary staff were still charged with the overall management of operations (in line with recommendation 4 of the Northumberland report). In the early stages of the outbreak the shortage of vets was made worse by their having to undertake non-veterinary work. Later in the outbreak, Regional Operations Directors were appointed thereby relieving veterinary staff of management responsibility for all non-veterinary tasks.

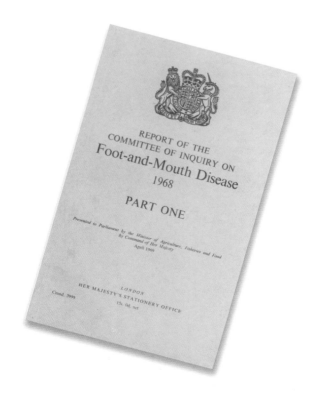

REPORT OF THE
COMMITTEE OF INQUIRY ON
Foot-and-Mouth Disease
1968

PART ONE

Presented to Parliament by the Minister of Agriculture, Fisheries and Food By Command of Her Majesty April 1969

LONDON
HER MAJESTY'S STATIONERY OFFICE
Cmnd. 3999
13s. 0d. net

■ *"Arrangements should be made to seek assistance from the armed services at an early stage. These arrangements should form part of the pre-outbreak planning and be at regional level (Part 2, Recommendation 50)."* The position on military assistance to the civil authorities has changed since the Northumberland Report of 1969. In particular, the standard arrangements which now exist for seeking assistance from the armed forces require that assistance should be sought on a national rather than a regional basis. Moreover, civil departments approaching the Ministry of Defence to request assistance from the armed services are expected to demonstrate that other avenues have been fully explored and exhausted. These procedures were followed in the 2001 outbreak and the Department considers that the Northumberland recommendation was applied as modified. However, contingency plans for foot and mouth disease did not consider the circumstances in which the armed services might be brought in, when this should be done or how they might assist. In 2001, the armed services became actively involved at the local level some three weeks after the outbreak once it became apparent to the Department that civilian contractors could not provide all the help required.

■ *"The Minister should be provided with adequate powers enabling him to take swift action to control foot and mouth disease; the powers should be sufficiently wide and flexible to enable him to deal with any disease situation (Part 2, Recommendation 102)."* This recommendation covered the re-enforcement of the powers applicable in 1967-68 as recommended elsewhere in the Northumberland report and was implemented. The Department dealt with the outbreak in 2001 under powers set out in the Animal Health Act 1981, which proved sufficient to eradicate the disease, and which for example covered the contiguous premises cull and the three kilometre cull, where animals had been exposed to infection. As the 2001 outbreak evolved, it became apparent to the Department that some areas would benefit from further reinforcement, in particular powers to slaughter animals to prevent the spread of disease, without the animals necessarily having to have been exposed to the disease. In addition, Ministers favoured clearer powers of entry to farms and new powers to vary compensation payable to farmers according to biosecurity standards. The Government is currently seeking these powers through an Animal Health Bill.

Drummond report on preparedness within the State Veterinary Service

2.38 In 1998-99 a working group, comprising state veterinary staff, examined the preparedness of the State Veterinary Service to deal with animal disease outbreaks. The group was chaired by Mr Richard Drummond, Head of Veterinary Services, Northern Region. He reported in February 1999. The report found considerable variation throughout the Service in the readiness to deal with outbreaks of exotic notifiable diseases, including foot and mouth. Existing contingency plans in many areas had not been updated because of other priorities and limited resources. In addition, a high turnover of administrative staff, and the resignation or retirement of experienced veterinary and technical staff had impaired the Service's ability to react.

2.39 The Drummond report expressed concern that with 'the speed at which foot and mouth disease might spread, the State Veterinary Service's resources could quickly become overwhelmed, particularly if a number of separate outbreaks occurred in separate locations at the same time'. It recommended enhancing the arrangements to gear-up resources through establishing call-off contracts for supplies, reaching understandings with Regional Service Centres for the loan of administrative staff, and approaching the Royal College of Veterinary Surgeons to maintain a list of retired vets who might be drawn upon to tackle an outbreak.

2.40 The report made the point that there was little time to debate the various options available for dealing with an outbreak once disease had broken out. The State Veterinary Service needed to clear its lines with all interested parties well in advance. The report identified five key areas for action:

■ Making a generic emergency plan for foot and mouth available to each Animal Health Divisional Office to use if desired.

■ The formulation of regional and divisional training plans.

■ Preparing national guidance on overcoming the problems associated with the supply of services and materials in dealing with outbreaks.

■ Ensuring that up to date instructions were available on computer.

■ Discussing with the veterinary profession how to improve relations with private vets.

2.41 By July 2000 the Department had made progress on many of the key areas for action, including the provision of a model generic emergency plan for Animal Health Divisional Offices and guidance on overcoming problems associated with the supply of services and materials. The generic plan was based on a plan drawn up by the Strathclyde Emergencies Co-ordination Committee. However, the Chief Veterinary Officer expressed his concern that other key issues had not been resolved, some two years after they had been identified by the Drummond report. The Department had not had time to address fully the slaughter and disposal of carcasses, training of staff in preparedness for an outbreak, the updating of existing contingency plans, and epidemiological capacity to deal with investigations about the spread of the disease if there were an outbreak. The State Veterinary Service was faced with finite resources and a wide range of tasks and workload to address, which required the Service to prioritise its activities. International risk assessments conducted by the Food and Agriculture Organisation of the United Nations, the Institute for Animal Health and the European Union considered that the most likely source of any outbreak of foot and mouth disease in Europe would involve entry through the eastern borders of Europe. The Department considers that existing controls were in place and that its prioritisation of work based on all available information at the time was correct.

Sources of scientific advice

2.42 In 1997 the Office of Science and Technology set out the key principles applying to the development and presentation of scientific advice and policy making. These were updated in July 2000 as Guidelines 2000 and are consistent with the principles underlying the Government's drive for evidence-based policy. Its key messages were that departments should:

- think ahead and identify early the issues on which they need scientific advice;

- get a wide range of advice from the best sources, including the right balance of scientific disciplines; and

- publish the scientific advice and all relevant papers.

The Department informed us that similar principles had already been applied to procedures within the Department since 1967 and this review confirmed the validity of existing processes.

2.43 The report of the inquiry, chaired by Lord Phillips, into Bovine Spongiform Encephalopathy (BSE) was published in October 2000. The concerns about the BSE epidemic and the government's response to it which prompted the Phillips inquiry have no close parallel with the foot and mouth disease epidemic. However, in preparing for an outbreak of animal disease the report did advocate "rigour in policy-making and openness to external and dissenting sources of advice, with explicit and careful treatment of risk." The inquiry also advocated:

- effective contingency planning;

- close co-operation among different branches of government;

- clarity of roles and responsibilities; and

- openness, trust and effective communication within government and with the public.

2.44 The national contingency plan for foot and mouth disease does not refer to the sources of scientific advice for understanding or controlling the disease during an outbreak. During a crisis it would be important for the Department to identify quickly those issues on which they would need advice and the best sources of that advice. From the outset of the 2001 epidemic the Chief Veterinary Officer drew on the knowledge and expertise of staff in the Department and its agencies, such as the State Veterinary Service and at the Veterinary Laboratories Agency, as well as veterinary epidemiologists from home and abroad who had the appropriate experience. The Department also made use of existing contacts with the World Health Organisation, the Food and Agriculture Organisation, the European Commission for the Control of Foot-and-Mouth Disease, the Institute for Animal Health, the Scientific Veterinary Committee, and the Centre for Applied Microbiology and Research. The Chief Veterinary Officer also held regular meetings with senior representatives of the veterinary profession at which the disease and control methods were discussed. The Department told us that all of these contacts had been established and were in regular use prior to BSE and the Phillips Inquiry.

2.45 A wider group involving external and government department experts was set up by the Chief Scientific Adviser on 24 March 2001 at the request of the Prime Minister. This group (the Foot and Mouth Disease Science Group) comprised three teams of university-based epidemiological modellers (who had already been obtaining data from the Department), virologists,

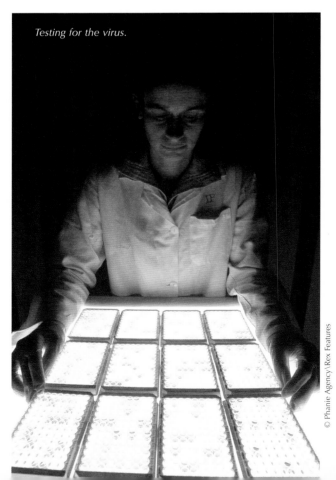

Testing for the virus.

vets and logisticians as well as a government veterinary epidemiologist. Advice from the Chief Scientific Adviser, which arose from discussion within this group, played a leading part in developing slaughter targets and other policies to control the epidemic after 24 March 2001.

2.46 The Foot and Mouth Disease Science Group was an informal group that was set up quickly, first meeting within two days of being formed. The Group included experts from a range of disciplines and much of the underlying research and projections has subsequently been publicised through media presentations and published papers. The Department's Chief Scientist at the time of the outbreak, who was a member of the Group, considers that it would have benefited from inclusion of a fuller range of sciences, for example, experts on the environmental and health consequences of options under consideration. Experts in these fields were represented, however, in the Joint Co-ordination Centre and the Cabinet Office Briefing Room.

2.47 The Phillips Inquiry also commented on what it saw as a deficiency in veterinary epidemiological expertise in the Department, recommending that provision should be made for training veterinarians in epidemiology[11]. The Department informed us that by the time the Phillips Inquiry reported it had:

- undertaken strategic recruiting and training - the epidemiology department at the Veterinary Laboratories Agency now comprises the largest group of postgraduate trained veterinary epidemiologists in the world, who are able to bring a range of expertise to epidemiological analyses;

- developed links with the University of Massey in New Zealand;

- funded a fellowship in veterinary epidemiology at Liverpool University; and

- asked epidemiologists at the Veterinary Laboratories Agency to design and run a MSc course with academic colleagues.

2.48 At the start of the 2001 outbreak, a Veterinary Epidemiology Unit was set up, comprising a headquarters team and field teams in the regions. A number of the epidemiologists came from overseas state veterinary services and scientific organisations including, by 26 February 2001, four from New Zealand. By late March 2001, the headquarters team comprised eight specialists, supported by five administrative staff; and in the field there were 15 epidemiological veterinary officers. At its peak the Unit had 45 staff. The Department considers that permanent veterinary officers of the State Veterinary Service would have understood general epidemiological principles from their other work, for example, on Bovine Spongiform Encephalopathy (BSE) and bovine

tuberculosis. Many had also attended a foot and mouth disease epidemiology course and others had obtained experience during the outbreak of classical swine fever in 2000 (see below). Even so, there was a need for more trained epidemiologists during the outbreak and the shortage meant that activities had to be carefully targeted, with field epidemiologists moving quickly from region to region as new disease hotspots developed.

Report on the classical swine fever outbreak in East Anglia in 2000

2.49 Classical swine fever is a disease that affects pigs. It spreads quickly and in some respects is similar in nature to foot and mouth disease. In 2000 there was an outbreak of classical swine fever in East Anglia. It affected 16 pig holdings; the first case was recorded on 4 August 2000 and the last on 3 November 2000. The disease was 'stamped out' by a policy of slaughter, backed by movement controls and biosecurity measures similar to those used to combat foot and mouth disease. Some 74,000 pigs were slaughtered and over 500 personnel were involved in dealing with the outbreak at some point. Vets from Ireland, the Netherlands and the United States assisted in eradicating the disease.

2.50 In October 2000 a project team comprising state vets was set up to consider and report on the response to the outbreak of classical swine fever. The project team reported in January 2001. It found that although the disease was successfully eradicated, the epidemic highlighted a number of problems in the Department's arrangements for disease control. For example, there were strong concerns about the effectiveness of:

- *Information Technology.* It was felt that, if there was a disease outbreak which required the setting up of more than one local Disease Control Centre, existing information systems would collapse.

- *Communications both internal and external.* Communications throughout the swine fever outbreak were reported to be a constant problem and it was difficult to communicate effectively with all those that needed to be kept informed.

- *Roles and responsibilities of staff.* A clearer definition of veterinary and administrative roles was needed.

- *The level of preparedness.* Disease control practices and the arrangements for notifying industry and other outside interests needed to be brought up to date.

---

11 *The study of the causes, occurrence, severity, distribution and control of disease.*

2.51 A number of lessons learned from the successful eradication of classical swine fever were implemented immediately in the fight against foot and mouth disease:

■ the involvement of stakeholders at local and national levels;

■ the management of the national Departmental Emergency Control Centre;

■ the development of local Disease Control Centres - 80 per cent of the State Veterinary Service's veterinary and technical staff and 25 per cent of its administrative staff had spent time on detached duty dealing with classical swine fever;

■ the organisation and use of Head Office and field epidemiology teams; and

■ the use of Geographical Information System for providing mapping support and graphical representation of the outbreak.

2.52 The Department also proposed to incorporate the lessons learned from the classical swine fever outbreak into a 'national emergency response plan'. There would be reviews of State Veterinary Service contingency planning, communications, information technology, and roles and responsibilities of staff. However, the foot and mouth disease outbreak began before this review process could begin and time did not allow for the introduction of new working practices in these areas.

Stakeholders were not formally consulted in preparing contingency plans

2.53 A serious outbreak of animal disease requires co-operation among a number of government departments, including those responsible for the environment, public health, transport, the armed services, the countryside and tourism. It also places responsibilities upon a range of public authorities: for example, local authority trading standards for licensing certain livestock movements, dealing with contraventions of legislation and the enforcement of illegal movements; the environment agencies for approving disposal methods and burial sites; and the police for assisting local authorities in enforcing movement restrictions, tasks which these organisations routinely carry out. It is important that all interested parties are fully aware of what is expected of them. Public authorities have a duty to be aware of their regulatory responsibilities.

2.54 Any strategy for dealing with the disease and its wider impacts depends for its success on the active co-operation of those closely affected and the wider acceptance of public opinion at large. However, the national contingency plan and veterinary instructions for foot and mouth disease were prepared by the Department without consultation with other key stakeholders, including other government departments, local authorities and representatives of key groups such as farmers and the veterinary profession. Some of these organisations were nevertheless involved in simulation exercises for animal disease control.

2.55 The national contingency plan for foot and mouth disease was publicly available but this fact was not publicised and it did not appear on the Department's website. This meant that awareness of its existence before the outbreak, and what it contained, was low. We found that key organisations, such as the Local Government Association, the National Farmers' Union, and representatives of livestock interests, either believed that the Department had no plans for dealing with an outbreak of foot and mouth disease, or had not seen them. We noted by comparison that other countries' contingency plans, such as Australia's Ausvetplan, were available on the Internet before the outbreak in Britain. Nevertheless, the Australian authorities have felt the need to revise their contingency plan as a result of the outbreak in the United Kingdom.

2.56 At the local level, other agencies were involved to varying degrees in preparing contingency plans. The Drummond report noted that in some areas, such as in Wales, the State Veterinary Service had participated in a multi-agency approach to disease control. In other parts of Britain, however, liaison with other agencies on disease control measures had deteriorated.

2.57 In Scotland we found that, in addition to the national contingency plan and local contingency plans developed at divisional level, the local councils in the affected areas had a well developed emergency planning approach. In Dumfries and Galloway, this had grown from experiences following the Lockerbie air disaster. Dumfries and Galloway Council initiated its Major Emergency Scheme on 28 February 2001, following possible identification of the disease in Scotland. Scottish Borders Council set up a helpline on 4 March 2001 following the first case in Dumfries and Galloway and activated its emergency plan quickly after the emergence of the disease in Newcastleton in late March 2001.

Contingency plans were tested to different degrees on a local basis

2.58 To be effective the planning for an outbreak of foot and mouth disease needs to be supported by training and exercises which simulate how an outbreak might develop on the ground. Such simulation exercises might involve the tracing of animal movements, staffing and running a control centre, epidemiology, and other aspects of the response to a disease outbreak. Simulation exercises are particularly important because of the long intervals that have occurred between disease outbreaks in the United Kingdom. Before the 2001 outbreak, few of the Department's staff would have had direct experience of a foot and mouth epidemic.

2.59 The State Veterinary Service held simulation exercises for animal disease control (not necessarily in respect of foot and mouth disease) at regular intervals during the last five years. Between 1995 and 1999 the United Kingdom held 84 simulation exercises - more than any other country in the European Union (**Figure 22**). The exercises varied in scope from desk exercises which focused on particular aspects of handling disease outbreaks, such as tracing the movement and location of animals, to field exercises involving a simulated disease outbreak and subsequent actions. During this same period, as well as handling its routine work, the State Veterinary Service also dealt with bovine tuberculosis and an outbreak of Newcastle disease in poultry, investigated 32,000 cases of Bovine Spongiform Encephalopathy (BSE) and traced and culled 60,000 cattle at risk from BSE. The last major disease control contingency exercise before the 2001 outbreak was held in Ayr in 1999. It involved staff from a wide range of organisations, including the State Veterinary Service, the Scottish Executive, the Scottish Environment Protection Agency, local and water authorities and the police.

2.60 The frequency and quality of the simulation exercises carried out in Britain varied between Animal Health Divisional Offices. The Drummond report found that opinion was divided within Animal Health Divisional Offices as to the usefulness of training exercises. Some staff had found the exercises useful in stimulating them to think about their role. Others considered that the exercises were not realistic and did not test contingency plans to their limit. Generally, however, the exercises were seen as helpful in reinforcing theoretical training, though they could not simulate fully the pressures that would exist in a real situation or the long-term commitment that would be needed. In these respects the outbreak of classical swine fever in 2000 referred to above provided much valuable, practical experience for those staff who were on the front line.

2.61 The Department told us that the involvement of local authorities in simulation exercises varied widely. Not all Animal Health Divisional Offices invited local authorities to contingency exercises. Where they were invited, often the response was poor or only junior officers attended.

22 | **Simulation exercises for animal disease control in the European Union, 1995 to 1999**

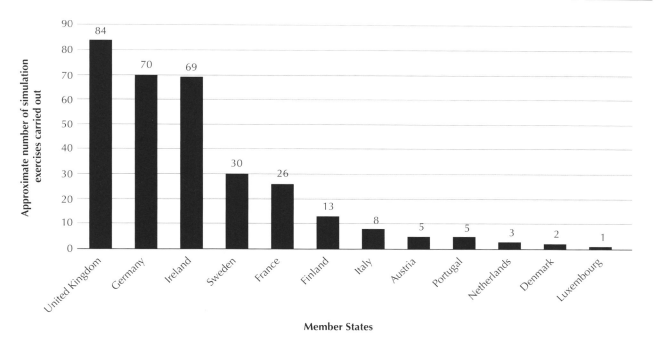

Member States

NOTES

1. Animal disease means an Office Internationale des Epizooties 'List A' disease, which includes foot and mouth disease.

2. Belgium and Greece did not carry out simulation exercises during this period as they experienced outbreaks of a List A disease. No simulation exercises are shown for Spain, but in each of the years between 1997 and 1999 immediate alerts were made when serious threats occurred.

Source: European Commission data supplied to the Department in March 2000.

The Department is revising its contingency plans for foot and mouth disease

2.62 In March 2002 the Department issued a draft interim contingency plan for the operational response to any future outbreak of foot and mouth disease (**Figure 23**). Similar work is being undertaken in Scotland and Wales. The draft, which codifies experience gained from the 2001 outbreak, has been discussed with stakeholder organisations and has been made available for wider discussion. It is available on the Department's website. The plan follows guidance published by the Cabinet Office's Civil Contingencies Secretariat, which was set up in July 2001, and the Department's own Emergencies Unit.

2.63 The Department is also working to revise and update existing local contingency plans and veterinary guidance and to ensure that they fit with the new interim operational plans. The plans taken together will aim to ensure that at the outset disease control is set within the context of its impact on the rural economy and the need to protect the environment and human health. The plans will be based on several assumptions that were developed during the 2001 outbreak as the most effective way of stamping out foot and mouth disease. The assumptions will be subject to veterinary risk assessment in the event of an outbreak to ensure that the response is proportionate.

2.64 The Department envisages that the revised contingency plans will be regularly tested at both local and national levels through simulation exercises involving the key personnel identified in the plans. The plan will also be revised and amended as necessary in the light of the recommendations of the Lessons Learned and Royal Society Inquiries.

23   **Key features of the Department's interim contingency plan**

The interim contingency plan does not seek to pre-empt the results of official inquiries and will be reviewed once their findings have been made public. The plan codifies lessons learned during the 2001 foot and mouth outbreak. It is a temporary measure, dealing solely with operational issues. The current Great Britain foot and mouth contingency plan has been in existence for many years and has been regularly updated. The plan was approved by the European Commission in 1993. The interim contingency plan was presented for discussion on 12 March 2002 and placed on the Department's website. A consultative meeting with stakeholders took place on the same day and another on 20 March 2002.

Details of the plan

1. The plan is split into sections outlining structures, lines of communication, roles and responsibilities at both national and local levels.

2. An alert system is outlined describing actions that need to be taken upon report of a suspected case (amber alert) and upon confirmation of disease (red alert).

3. The response to the disease alert would be controlled using the recognised Gold, Silver and Bronze Command structure (Gold - Strategic, Silver - Tactical, Bronze - Operational).

4. At a national level there is consideration of the role of a Joint Co-ordination Centre, a Disease Emergency Control Centre, a Foot and Mouth Disease Programme Board and a Co-ordination Committee (or perhaps the Cabinet Office Briefing Room).

5. Use is made of a technique called process mapping to define initial action and responsibilities.

6. Further detail is provided on issues such as: resources, training, accommodation, information technology, procurement, stores, disposal, serology, financial, accounting and management information, communications, publicity and disease awareness, stakeholder involvement, vaccination, health and safety, and contingency testing.

7. The plan provides job descriptions for key personnel (such as Regional Operations Directors) at both national and local levels.

8. Further information provides detail on the relationship with the devolved administrations at an operational level, personal biosecurity protocols, transport specifications, daily situation reports, key personnel contacts, and foot and mouth stock lists held at Animal Health Offices.

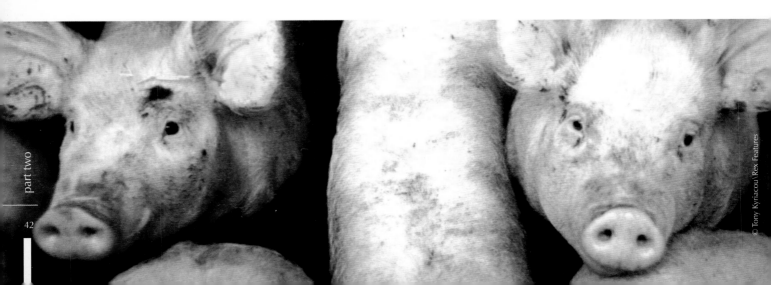

© Tony Kyriacou/Rex Features

Part 3

Handling the outbreak

3.1 Prompt and effective action at the outset is vital if an outbreak of foot and mouth disease is to be quickly contained and eradicated so as to keep its impact to a minimum. Success is only likely to be achieved if everyone involved, the Department and stakeholders, knows what is required of them and are kept fully informed.

3.2 This Part of the Report examines the Department's handling of the foot and mouth epidemic in 2001 and how quickly and effectively it was brought under control. We found that:

■ foot and mouth disease was eradicated quickly in some areas (paragraphs 3.4 to 3.10);

■ those involved worked extremely hard to bring the epidemic under control (paragraphs 3.11 to 3.12); and

■ there were severe problems in handling the outbreak in the worst-hit areas (paragraph 3.13 onwards).

3.3 Given the extent of initial 'seeding' of the disease and the unprecedented nature and scale of the outbreak, the Department faced a monumental task to eradicate the disease. Despite, as noted in Part 2, the scale of the epidemic overwhelming the Department's preparations, the Department and its partners responded with application and commitment. The Department also made adaptations to its plans as the pattern of the outbreaks emerged. These efforts enabled the disease to be eradicated quickly in some areas and prevented its spread to high risk pig and dairy farming areas. The Department made a number of judgements in handling the disease - such as when to introduce a national movement ban on livestock movements or to call in outside assistance - which with hindsight would have been different. It must be recognised, however, that the Department was under considerable pressure from the start of the outbreak and had to make its judgements on the basis of the information available and changing and sometimes contradictory evidence. Decisions had to be taken quickly and it was inevitable that in retrospect some of these would have been different.

Foot and mouth disease was eradicated quickly in some areas

3.4 The disease was eradicated relatively quickly in some areas. In the Infected Areas covered by half of the 18 Disease Control Centres, the time between confirmation of the first and last infected premises was 62 days or less (**Figure 24 overleaf**). The disease had in fact been 'stamped out' by mid-April 2001 in most parts of central and eastern England. Outbreaks were also brought quite quickly under control in Anglesey and southern Scotland. In both these areas, there was rigorous culling of exposed animals on farms around infected premises.

3.5 In other areas, such as Cumbria, the North East, North Yorkshire, Devon, Lancashire, Staffordshire and parts of Wales, the outbreaks took longer to eradicate. These outbreaks continued into June 2001 and beyond, with flare-ups around certain 'hotspots'. In Cumbria and the North East the epidemic lasted for seven months, from February until September 2001. However, the interval between first and last confirmed cases in parts of these larger areas was much less. The outbreak in Allendale in Northumberland in August 2001 was after a period of 12 weeks with no cases in the North East and lasted 34 days.

3.6 These variations between different areas arose from a number of factors, including:

■ the extent of initial disease 'seeding' - this was particularly extensive, for example, in Cumbria, in Northumberland and in Devon. In Cumbria, subsequent epidemiological investigations have established that at least 38 farms were infected before the first case was confirmed on 1 March 2001. In Devon, the first confirmed case involved a sheep dealer with 13 separate livestock premises.

■ the speed of discovery of the source case in the area and the extent of prior warning;

24 **Time to eradicate the disease by Disease Control Centre**

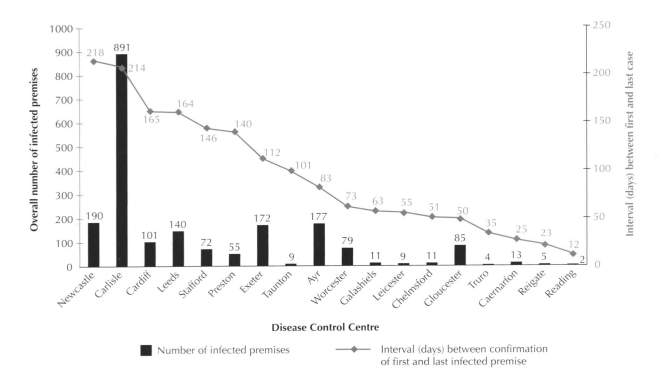

Number of infected premises

Interval (days) between confirmation of first and last infected premise

NOTES

1. This figure shows the cases handled by each local Disease Control Centre. Where there were outbreaks of disease on the edge of a county covered by a Disease Control Centre, for example, Cumbria, which was covered by Carlisle, the outbreak was sometimes handled by a neighbouring Disease Control Centre. This explains the differences that appear between the figures shown here (and in Appendix 7) and those cited for counties in paragraph 1.10.

2. The elapsed time for Newcastle includes more than 30 cases which were dealt with jointly by the Carlisle Disease Control Centre and Newcastle area office, before a stand-alone Disease Control Centre was set up in Newcastle on 30 March 2001.

3. We show time to eradication for Disease Control Centres. In practice, a Disease Control Centre sometimes tackled several distinct outbreaks within the area it covered. For example, the Cardiff Disease Control Centre, with an area office at Llandrindod Wells, handled clusters of cases in north and south Powys and the South Wales valleys.

Source: National Audit Office analysis of data in the Department's Disease Control System.

- comparative livestock densities and local farming practices - disease control was easier in areas such as the Cheshire plains, where farms were held in compact units, than in areas such as Allendale in Northumberland and Settle in North Yorkshire, where farmers' livestock was dispersed across scattered parcels of land;

- the level of support received from local stakeholders, including farmers and local agencies, and the level of compliance with local disease control measures and biosecurity advice and guidance;

- the number and nature of resources available to fight the disease; and

- the level of preparedness.

3.7 Responses improved as local offices built up experience of fighting the disease. This is demonstrated, for example, by the efficiency of the actions taken by the Exeter control centre when faced by a local flare-up around Clayhanger in mid-June 2001 (**Figure 25**).

3.8 The Department did well to contain the disease substantially within those areas where infection was confirmed during the first three weeks of the epidemic. The disease was kept out of much of East Anglia, the East Midlands, southern England, west Wales and central and northern Scotland. This protected a number of important dairy and pig farming areas. The outbreak could have been much more extensive if the disease had been allowed to spread to the pig areas, as pigs are major shedders of the virus, especially in exhaled air.

25 | **'Clayhanger'- an example of efficient disease control**

On 11 June 2001 an outbreak of disease was confirmed in Clayhanger, an area straddling the Devon/Somerset border and at a distance from any earlier infected premises. The source case was a sheep flock in which there had been longstanding infection. Poor biosecurity and a large number of movements by owners between scattered holdings had contributed to local spread.

There was the potential for a major flare-up of the disease and the infection of neighbouring areas. The Department responded promptly, benefiting from logistical arrangements set up by the Military. The number of stock involved was considerable, over 500 cattle and 3,500 sheep on the infected premises and more than 8,000 animals (mainly sheep) on contiguous premises. The arrangements made for slaughter and disposal were effective, with slaughter carried out within 24 hours and disposal soon after. Carcasses were removed quickly from farms and taken to a collection centre for incineration or rendering. By 18 June 2001 this local outbreak, involving seven infected premises and 24 contiguous premises, had been stamped out.

3.9 The Department also did well in ensuring that once the disease had been stamped out in an area, it did not reappear. In 1967-68 the tail of the epidemic had been prolonged by a re-emergence of the disease during restocking of previously infected farms. Cleansing and disinfecting had been inadequate. In 2001, there were no cases of the disease re-emerging because of poor cleansing and disinfecting. A new outbreak occurred in August 2001 in the Allendale area of Northumberland and probably arose because of poor biosecurity. In spite of the rapid imposition of a Restricted Infected Area and rapid diagnosis and culling, there were still 32 cases mostly linked to the source farm.

3.10 In response to questions from the European Parliament's Temporary Committee on the 2001 outbreak of foot and mouth disease, the European Commission has stated that, "The Commission is in general satisfied with the implementation of Community and national measures by Member States. Nonetheless, there are clear lessons to be drawn from the outbreak. Member States have taken swift and decisive action to counteract foot and mouth disease in the European Union. This is reflected by the rapid recovery of 'foot and mouth disease-free without vaccination' status in France, the Netherlands, Ireland and the United Kingdom, in each case about three months after the last reported outbreak."

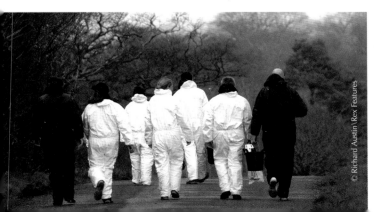

Those involved worked extremely hard to bring the epidemic under control

3.11 The disease was eradicated through the commitment and dedication of the Department's staff (vets, animal health and other field officers and administrators) and many others who assisted in the disease control campaign. Those in the field worked punishingly long days - some up to 14 days or more without a break - in stressful and often distressing conditions. Little leave was taken. Some staff also worked for long periods away from home. Many staff had to shoulder new responsibilities; and some field officers had to take part in activities that they may never have envisaged, such as holding livestock during slaughter. Similar punishing hours and conditions were endured by veterinary, policy, legal and administrative staff in the London offices of the Department.

3.12 Administrative staff also worked hard, often in cramped temporary portacabins. They had to adapt to rapidly changing circumstances and to assimilate and carry out many new instructions. Those from other parts of government, the voluntary sector, farmers and contractors also made a substantial contribution. The unremitting 'battle' against the disease caused substantial stress to many of those involved. In April 2001 a report on the Carlisle Disease Control Centre found that staff were suffering from a range of stress-related conditions, including exhaustion, disrupted sleep patterns, nightmares, loss of appetite, anger, frustration and a sense of powerlessness. Steps taken by local management addressed these problems, including ensuring that staff received appropriate training, took effective breaks from work, were provided with onsite welfare officers, and were given access to a 24 hour helpline.

There were severe problems in handling the outbreak in the worst-hit areas

3.13 The rest of this Part of the Report considers the problems that the Department faced in dealing with the outbreak, what the consequences were and how they were overcome. It examines:

- the organisational structures that had to be developed (paragraphs 3.14 to 3.23);

- the need for other agencies to become involved (paragraphs 3.24 to 3.32);

- the shortages of resources that had to be addressed (paragraphs 3.33 to 3.48);

Photograph shows vets, field staff and many others assisted in bringing the disease under control.

- the need for movement controls and strict biosecurity measures to contain the disease (paragraphs 3.49 to 3.63);

- the difficulties in identification (paragraphs 3.64 to 3.81), slaughter (paragraphs 3.82 to 3.94) and disposal (paragraphs 3.95 to 3.103) of infected or exposed animals; and

- the challenge of communicating effectively with those involved (paragraphs 3.104 to 3.110).

Organisational structures improved as the crisis developed

Initially operations were directed by the Department's veterinary officers

3.14 On 21 February 2001, within 24 hours of confirmation of disease, a national Departmental Emergency Control Centre (the 'DECC') was set up at the State Veterinary Service's headquarters in Page Street, London. The Chief Veterinary Officer had overall charge of disease control strategy. Disease Control Centres, responsible for operational activities relating to local disease control, were established once an infected premises was confirmed in a particular area. Most were established in or near Animal Health Divisional Offices and were typically up and running within 48 hours. Each was run by a Divisional Veterinary Manager, who oversaw local implementation of the national control strategy and was responsible for procurement and communications with stakeholders and the media.

3.15 In the report of a mission carried out in the United Kingdom between 12 and 16 March 2001, the European Commission commented on the impressive speed with which the Departmental Emergency Control Centre and local Disease Control Centres (the 'DCCs') had been established. Other bodies were more critical, however, of the Department's initial response to the outbreak. The National Farmers' Union told us that in the early stages the response suffered from a lack of co-ordination between vets and other Government staff. In some areas, such as Stafford, the management of responsibilities and the allocation of tasks had been handled well from the outset. In many areas, however, Divisional Veterinary Managers were overwhelmed by the scale and extraordinary demands of the managerial and organisational role that they would need to perform to ensure that resources were deployed effectively.

From mid-March 2001 new structures were developed

3.16 The Prime Minister and Cabinet were kept closely informed of the developing situation and the progress made in controlling the disease. Until the tracing of many of the sheep that had passed through livestock markets before 23 February 2001 had been completed, the potential scale of the epidemic remained uncertain.

On 4 March 2001, by which date there were 69 confirmed outbreaks, the Department advised that the "likely course of the disease would become clear shortly and that it could possibly peak by the end of the week".

3.17 By 12 March 2001, however, as more data became available from the field, the Department's epidemiological modelling team had established a good representation of the epidemic and predicted that confirmed cases would rise steeply, so that by early April 2001 there would be more than 1,600 detected infected premises and many more undetected. The Minister of Agriculture and the Chief Veterinary Officer informed the Prime Minister that the country was facing a very large outbreak of between 1,000 and 2,000 cases. It had also become clear to the Department by mid-March 2001 that the size of the outbreak was placing impossibly heavy demands on the resources, management and organisational capacity of the State Veterinary Service. On 14 March 2001, facing the danger of a breakdown in the field, the Department appointed the chief executive of the Intervention Board to direct logistical operations at the Department's headquarters in Page Street. The key stages in the organisational response are shown in **Figure 26**.

3.18 From 19 March 2001 onwards, senior administrators, mostly of Grades 3 and 5 level, were sent to the main Disease Control Centres as Regional Operations Directors. They relieved Divisional Veterinary Managers of some of the burden of local external communications and organised logistical and administrative support, including the slaughter and disposal of affected animals. They also drove forward improvements in resource organisation and management. The National Farmers' Union told us that the appointment of Regional Operations Directors greatly improved local organisation and that this should have happened earlier.

3.19 At the beginning of the outbreak the Department took the lead in directing and co-ordinating the Government's response to the outbreak. The Prime Minister was closely engaged, receiving regular briefings and holding meetings with Ministers, the farming industry and wider rural interests. Once the national scale of the outbreak became clear, the Prime Minister with the Cabinet and the Minister of Agriculture oversaw the development of policy. The Cabinet Office chaired meetings of officials from the first week and in the early stages organised several meetings of an ad hoc Ministerial Committee on foot and mouth disease. On 22 March 2001 the Cabinet Office Briefing Room was opened and until September 2001 oversaw disease strategy and operations but not policy. It was chaired initially usually by the Prime Minister or the Secretary of State for Defence and later by the Department's Ministers. Its small secretariat serviced daily meetings of ministers from a range of affected departments.

26 Timeline of the organisational response

Date in 2001	Cumulative number of infected premises	Development
20 February	1	The first outbreak, in Essex, is confirmed.
21 February	2	A National Departmental Emergency Disease Control Centre is set up in Page Street, London, along with a Veterinary Epidemiological Unit, to analyse outbreaks, and an Epidemiological Modelling Team, to predict the epidemic's likely scale and advise on control measures. A Disease Control Centre is set up in Chelmsford.
23 February	6	The source case is identified in Northumberland.
25 February	7	The first case is confirmed in Devon, highlighting the long-distance spread caused by livestock marketing.
2 March	38	A Veterinary Risk Assessment Unit is established, to prepare assessments on the risks of agricultural and rural activities.
6 March	80	A Disease Control System database is set up.
12 March	187	Tracing and internal modelling evidence indicates a 'very large' outbreak.
14 March	219	A Director of Foot and Mouth Disease Operations is appointed. The Department agrees on the nature of the military's involvement with the Ministry of Defence.
19 March	352	Regional Operations Directors are appointed for Cumbria and Devon and, later, to other centres.
20 March	394	The foot and mouth crisis is made the top priority of the Cabinet Office.
22 March	479	The Cabinet Office Briefing Room is opened.
24 March	577	The Chief Scientist's Group is formed.
26 March	644	The Joint Co-ordination Centre begins work in Page Street and the Director of Foot and Mouth Disease Operations becomes the Director of the Joint Co-ordination Centre.

3.20 From 26 March 2001, the Cabinet Office was supported by a Joint Co-ordination Centre at the Department's Page Street headquarters in London. The Joint Co-ordination Centre was headed by the Director of Operations and supported by military and civilian deputies. Its objectives were to create and maintain an accurate ground picture, to create an all informed 'network' and to facilitate the passage of information flows, information management and dissemination of instructions. The Joint Co-ordination Centre performed three main roles:

■ it provided the Cabinet Office Briefing Room with daily information, worked out how decisions of the Cabinet Office Briefing Room could most effectively be implemented, and distributed information and instructions to Disease Control Centres;

■ it informed and co-ordinated the contribution from all government departments and other agencies; and

■ it established better co-ordination of military, veterinary and administrative resources at Disease Control Centres and promoted the exchange of good practice.

3.21 At the height of the crisis the Joint Co-ordination Centre operated seven days a week. It was modelled on the structure of a military operations room and was composed of a number of "cells", each with clear operational responsibility for a specific activity. To ensure co-ordination between policy and operations, briefings were provided three times a day on current progress and the major issues arising. The aim was to identify operational problems and issues and to task individuals to solve them. The Joint Co-ordination Centre was led by the Department's staff with representatives from a range of other Government departments and agencies, as well as the Association of Chief Police Officers, the National Farmers' Union and liaison officers from the devolved administrations in Scotland and Wales. By mid-April 2001 there were about 50 staff with desks in the Joint Co-ordination Centre including over 20 military personnel, and 60-70 staff would be present for the briefing meetings.

3.22 As well as advice from the Chief Veterinary Officer, the Cabinet Office Briefing Room drew on scientific advice from the Foot and Mouth Disease Science Group and other government departments.

The new arrangements improved the response to the disease

3.23 The new structures (**Figure 27**) addressed problems that had emerged during the first three weeks of the crisis. They improved the effectiveness of the disease response in four ways:

■ State vets were relieved of many tasks and given more time for veterinary work.

■ The Joint Co-ordination Centre helped to identify and overcome resource bottlenecks, particularly those affecting slaughter and disposal. For example, when captive bolt guns (required for safe and humane slaughter) were in short supply in late March 2001, the Joint Co-ordination Centre arranged for them to be imported and distributed to those centres in greatest need.

27   **Organisation of foot and mouth disease work from 26 March 2001**

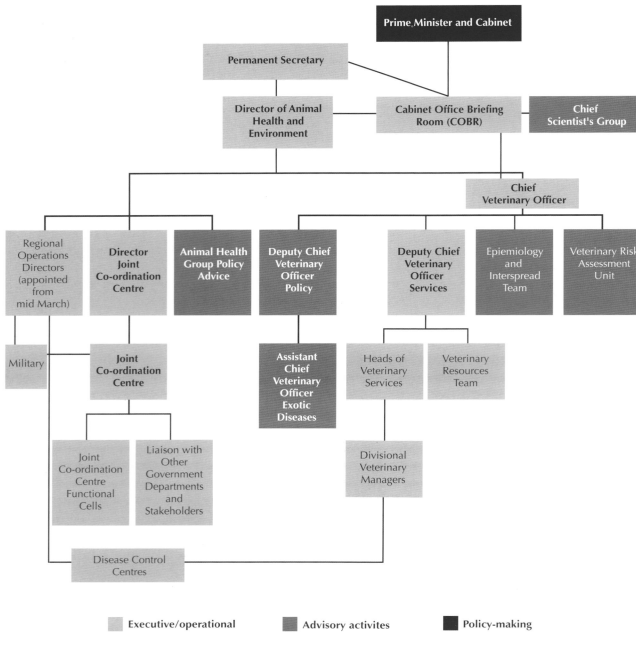

Executive/operational   Advisory activites   Policy-making

NOTE

Attendance at the Cabinet Office Briefing Room comprised Ministers and senior officials from all relevant Departments and Agencies.

Source: Department for Environment, Food and Rural Affairs

- Measures were taken to promote cross-agency co-ordination and to improve communications with stakeholders.

- More efficient operational structures were set up within Disease Control Centres.

It took time to get other agencies involved

The armed services became directly involved in mid-March 2001

3.24 The Department kept the military informed from the outset and had regular discussions, but did not call for large-scale assistance until mid-March 2001 (**Figure 28**). The Department had believed it could manage with the support of private contractors so long as the number of new cases was below 10 or so a day. By the second week of March 2001, however, the daily number of new confirmed cases had reached 20 and there were growing signs of a breakdown in the field. After discussion with the Ministry of Defence, the Department concluded that the assistance of the armed services in logistics planning at all operational levels would be valuable and made arrangements to call the armed services in. On 14 March 2001 four military vets arrived and on 16 March an armed services logistics coordinator was assigned to Exeter, where the disposal problem was most acute. Between 19 and 22 March 2001, military units were deployed in Devon, Cumbria, Worcester and Dumfries, and subsequently in other areas. On 25 March 2001, armed services logistics experts moved into the Department's Page Street headquarters to help form the Joint Co-ordination Centre and to contribute to co-ordinating the operation on a national level.

3.25 Military support was provided as Military Aid to the Civil Authorities, and specifically within the subset of these procedures known as Military Aid to Other Government Departments. All Military Aid to the Civil Authorities is provided at the request of the civil authority. In the case of Military Aid to Other Government Departments, another government department asks the Ministry of Defence to undertake tasks for which it is responsible. Legally, a Defence Council Order is required to undertake a task falling under Military Aid to Other Government Departments. Support for all Military Aid to the Civil Authorities tasks is provided from within existing Ministry of Defence resources. The Ministry of Defence has no units designated for tasks under Military Aid to the Civil Authorities, units are not trained specifically for such tasks, and the Ministry of Defence is not funded for them. The Ministry of Defence provides support through the deployment of military capabilities available at the time and does not provide support if there is a credible civil alternative.

3.26 The armed services played a key supportive role, assisting centrally and locally in the organisational and logistical arrangements, particularly for slaughter, transport and disposal. The military's contribution was significant, both in terms of numbers and impact, and helped to 'turn the tide' in the battle against the disease. By 31 March 2001, 1,000 troops were deployed and numbers built up to a mid-April 2001 peak of around 2,100. From late May 2001, troops began to be withdrawn from some areas such as in Scotland, where the outbreak was believed to be under control.

28 **Chronology of the military's involvement in the 2001 outbreak**

Date in 2001	Cumulative number of infected premises	Development
20 February	1	The Department contacts the Armed Forces' Minister to warn of a possible future request for military assistance.
1 March	31	The Department formally notifies the Ministry of Defence that it is considering requesting military assistance.
7 March	99	The Department discusses with the Ministry of Defence possible uses of military resources, but concludes no help is needed, except Army marksmen to slaughter outdoor pigs. A request for the latter is made on 9 March.
14 March	219	The Department agrees on the need for military assistance and four military vets arrive. The Department meets the Ministry of Defence to agree on the nature of the military's involvement.
16 March	270	An armed services logistics co-ordinator is sent to Exeter and a senior Departmental official at the National Control Centre is assigned to co-ordinate assistance from the armed services.
19 March onwards	352	Military assistance is deployed in Devon, Cumbria, Worcester, Dumfries and Galloway, and elsewhere.
25 March	606	Armed services representatives arrive at the Department's Page Street headquarters.
26 March	644	The Joint Co-ordination Centre is set up with military involvement.

part three

3.27 Each brigade operated within the well-established regional military structure designed to meet national emergency situations, but worked according to the instructions of the Department's Regional Operations Directors. The military made a particular contribution in two important areas:

- **Improving organisation and lines of communications**. Control centre operations rooms were established along military lines, helping to add direction and drive to the disease control campaign.

- **Organising slaughter, transport and disposal logistics**. This involved identifying contractors and disposal sites and arranging transport. The logistical challenge was huge: at the height of the outbreak the daily weight of carcasses moved was over half the weight of the ammunition the armed services supplied during the entire Gulf War.

3.28 The Northumberland Inquiry into the outbreak of foot and mouth disease in 1967-68 said that it should not be necessary to wait until an outbreak is widespread before obtaining the assistance of military personnel. Circumstances could arise making it highly desirable to call on the armed services for some forms of assistance to control the disease even during the course of a single or small number of outbreaks. Speed and efficiency in slaughter of infected and in-contact animals, disposal of carcasses and disinfection of premises are the most vital elements in controlling an outbreak and these will not be achieved without disciplined workers under experienced and trained supervisors. The Northumberland report went on to note that, after the 1967-68 epidemic, there had been negotiations between the then Ministry of Agriculture and the Ministry of Defence that in outbreaks of foot and mouth disease any of the Ministry's regional controllers or the Deputy Director of the Veterinary Field Service in Scotland could approach Army Commands as soon as they considered that all suitable civilian labour resources had been committed. This agreement allowed them to recommend that in a future outbreak arrangements should be made to seek assistance from the armed forces at an early stage.

3.29 The Government's internal report on military involvement in 1967-68 advised that "the earlier the military can be called in the better". As noted above, currently military support is provided at the national level. Contact with the Ministry of Defence was initiated on day 1 of the 2001 outbreak and by 14 March 2001 it was apparent that the logistic and organisational capability of the armed forces would be of value. The Department told us that in 2001 it did not call for large-scale military assistance until three weeks into the outbreak because the Government considered that the early stages of the epidemic presented no obvious requirement for military participation. Many of the stakeholders and agencies we consulted felt that the deployment of troops had had a very positive impact in helping to control the disease and that the armed services should have been called in much earlier.

The speed with which other bodies became involved varied

3.30 The scale and impact of the epidemic meant that other government departments and agencies, local authorities, voluntary organisations and stakeholders were affected and had an important role to play in helping to combat the disease. The Department began liaising with other government departments, agencies and local authorities on day 1 of the outbreak. The first national stakeholders' meeting was held on 23 February 2001 at which point six cases had been confirmed. On 25 February 2001 the Environment Agency's incident room opened and the Department and the Agency issued a joint statement on the disposal of carcasses. On 27 February 2001, by which time 16 cases had been confirmed, local authorities were given powers to close rights of way and representatives of the devolved administrations were posted to the Department's Page Street headquarters

3.31 Some organisations felt that the Department was slow to recognise the full extent of the role they could play in combating the disease. Although some organisations, such as the Institute for Animal Health and the Veterinary Laboratories Agency, were involved from the start, other bodies told us that they were surprised that they had not been involved earlier. The Local Government Association told us that more should have been done to draw quickly on the services, skills and knowledge of local authorities. And North Yorkshire County Council, for example, was critical of the lack of prior consultation on the operation to deal with the foot and mouth outbreak.

3.32 In Dumfries and Galloway the Council Emergency Centre, which had sophisticated communication facilities and desks for key partners such as the police, fire service and contractors, was established quickly and placed at the disposal of the Divisional Veterinary Manager. Similarly in Wales, the close involvement of the National Assembly helped to mobilise local resources.

There were difficulties in getting sufficient human resources

'We had a major problem with staffing… we ran out of vets; we did not have enough technical staff; we had to train people to bleed animals; we had to find administrative staff and even drawing on other government departments we have had a serious resource problem' Mr James Scudamore, Chief Veterinary Officer, speaking on 31 October 2001 before the Select Committee on Environment, Food and Rural Affairs

3.33 On the eve of the outbreak, the Animal Health Divisional Offices of England, Scotland and Wales had 900 staff. By mid-April 2001, at the outbreak's height, around 1,200 vets and 7,000 administrative and field support staff were engaged in disease eradication at

Disease Control Centres. They were supported by more than 2,000 soldiers and an additional 'army' of slaughterers, valuers and employees of contractors and government bodies and agencies. This build up of resources was impressive. During the early weeks, however, resources were severely stretched. Shortages of resources contributed to delays in identification, slaughter and disposal.

The Department overcame a severe shortage of vets

3.34 In its 1991 guidelines the European Commission had described vets as 'the resource factor most critical to effective disease control'. Vets played a key role in diagnosing disease, overseeing slaughter arrangements and providing advice to farmers and others. With their training, experience and knowledge of the Department's systems and regulations, state vets formed the backbone of the disease response and performed key managerial and strategic roles in Disease Control Centres.

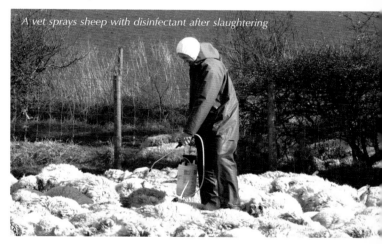

A vet sprays sheep with disinfectant after slaughtering

3.35 On the eve of the outbreak, there were 213 veterinary officers[12] in the State Veterinary Service. Numbers were seven per cent below complement, mainly because of recruitment difficulties in South East England. In addition to these state vets, the Department was able at the start of the outbreak to call on the services of 117 Temporary Veterinary Inspectors who were already working with the Department. The temporary vets were paid on a daily basis and worked under the Department's direction. In the private sector there were also around 7,000 Local Veterinary Inspectors, who, during their normal practice work, were paid by the Department for carrying out Departmental duties. During the crisis, some of these volunteered to become Temporary Veterinary Inspectors, while others carried out movement licence checks on the livestock of non-infected farms.

3.36 During the early weeks of the 2001 outbreak, many Disease Control Centres experienced severe shortages of vets and this affected disease control. The Chief Veterinary Officer admitted that at the height of the outbreak the Department "simply ran out of vets". In

12 Full-time equivalents

mid-March 2001, inspectors from the European Union's Food and Veterinary Office were told that vets were working at full stretch, having to visit and examine stock on up to 10 holdings a day.

3.37 The veterinary resources available to the Department were built up from just over 300 (including Temporary Veterinary Inspectors) in late February 2001 to around 1,600 in May 2001 **(Figure 29)**. But until April 2001 the growth in the number of vets lagged behind the growth in the number of infected premises **(Figure 30)**. Work on infected premises - involving examining livestock and diagnosis, taking samples, the serving of restrictions, advising on biosecurity and supervising slaughter - was

only one aspect of vets' workload. Vets were also involved in patrol visits to at risk farms, in following up tracings, in checking that on-farm preliminary cleansing and disinfecting were satisfactory, in sero-surveillance[13] and in work connected with movement licences.

3.38 The Department addressed veterinary shortages by: (i) drawing on agreed standby arrangements to obtain 50 vets from the Veterinary Laboratories Agency and other parts of government; (ii) borrowing nearly 600 vets from overseas state veterinary services, mostly from signatories to an International Veterinary Reserve Agreement (Australia, Canada, Ireland and New Zealand) and from the United States, in response to a

29 **Numbers of vet available for foot and mouth disease work[1], weeks 1-12 of the epidemic**

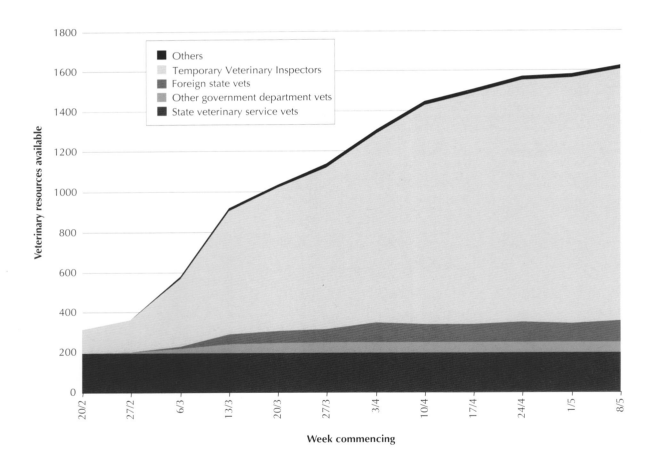

NOTES

1. The numbers of Temporary Veterinary Inspectors working at any given point in time was much lower. For example, in mid-April 2001 around 1,500 vets were available but only around 1,200 were working for the Department. In early May 2001, the ratio was lower, at around 1,000 out of 1,600. The differences arise because data are for those appointed and on the Department's 'books' whereas private practices typically registered several vets as 'available' but supplied them in rotation; some vets worked for the Department for only several days a month and others needed periodic breaks.

2. We have assumed in this figure that 200 of the State Veterinary Service's 213 field vets were regularly on foot and mouth disease duty during the crisis: even at the peak of the crisis, not all Animal Health Divisions in Britain had an outbreak to deal with.

Source: National Audit Office analysis of the Department's data

13 *Sero-surveillance involves the collection of serum from a sample of animals to be tested in a laboratory for evidence of injection.*

request made to them by the Chief Veterinary Officer on 23 February 2001; and (iii) recruiting more than 2,500 Temporary Veterinary Inspectors from private practices and locum agencies. In addition, from 19 March 2001, vets were relieved of many non-veterinary tasks, following the appointment of Regional Operations Directors. These measures were effective so that, by mid-April 2001, the Department had the number of vets it felt were needed to contain the outbreak.

3.39 Temporary Veterinary Inspectors provided the great bulk of the Department's veterinary field-force during the epidemic. Their recruitment was more difficult than had been expected, however. By the third week of the outbreak, around 300 Temporary Veterinary Inspectors had responded to local and national appeals. Evidence from surveys of veterinary practices suggested that others were deterred by what they saw as the low rate of remuneration of £160 a day, although this was the established rate in respect of foot and mouth disease work before the outbreak.

3.40 In the early stages of the outbreak the Chief Veterinary Officer advised the Minister of Agriculture that veterinary shortages were "posing a major constraint on disease control". On 20 March 2001, the Prime Minister told the Department that the shortage needed to be resolved urgently and that it should "offer what was needed" to recruit more Temporary Veterinary Inspectors . On 21 March 2001, following discussions with the British Veterinary Association, a new higher daily rate of £250 was agreed, backdated to the start of the crisis. The Department also relaxed the age limit requirement, which had initially meant that only vets aged below 65 could apply.

3.41 Helped by a high profile recruitment campaign, these changes led to a sharp rise in applications: by early April 2001 more than 1,000 Temporary Veterinary Inspectors were registered with the Department; and by early May 2001 there were more than 1,200. During the outbreak, more than 2,500 additional Temporary Veterinary Inspectors were recruited, most working, on average, for around eight weeks. Around a hundred were aged 65 or over. For more than 200 of the vets, English was a second language and this occasionally led to communication difficulties with farmers.

30   **Comparison of number of vets working and number of infected premises confirmed between March and May 2001**

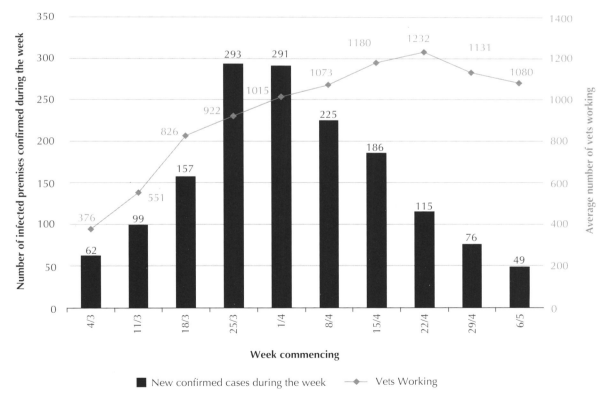

NOTE

As explained in the note to Figure 29, adjustments have been made to the Department's data for the early weeks to take account of the fact that some private vets, who were registered with the Department as Temporary Veterinary Inspectors, worked for only certain periods of each month.

Source: National Audit Office analysis of the Department's data.

3.42 Effective veterinary resources were increased further by relaxing the quarantine protocols for vets after visiting infected premises. From 10 March 2001, following advice from the Institute for Animal Health, the interval a vet had to wait before being able to investigate a further report of suspected infection was reduced from five days to 72 hours. On 30 March 2001 the Department reduced the interval from 72 hours to 24 hours. For areas such as Cumbria, which faced particular pressures, the interval was reduced further on 17 April 2001 from 24 hours to overnight providing rigorous biosecurity measures had been followed.

The Department faced challenges in recruiting support and administrative staff

3.43 The contribution of animal health officers and administrative support staff was crucial. Animal health officers helped vets during on-farm visits and oversaw the subsequent disposal and cleansing operations. They also assisted in the blood sampling of animals. Administrative support staff dealt with movement licenses, transport and accommodation, resource allocation and financial matters. They all worked under severe pressure.

3.44 During the early months of the crisis, some Disease Control Centres reported acute shortages of animal health officers, administrative staff and experienced managers. It was difficult to recruit animal health officers with the appropriate skills and many administrative staff were seconded for only short periods from other government departments. In most Animal Health Divisions, there were no pre-outbreak agreements with other government bodies to draw in such staff during an emergency and there were no international stand by arrangements for animal health officers to be loaned by overseas state veterinary services. The shortages meant that staff had an enormous workload in monitoring activities of contractors, slaughterers and armed services personnel. It also resulted in vets being required to carry out non-veterinary tasks; and there were some delays in processing invoices and licences to move animals.

3.45 Additional staff were obtained from other departments and agencies and by direct recruitment from the private sector. By April 2001 the number of animal health officers had increased fourfold to over 800. The increase in administrative support and general field staff was even more dramatic, from 500 to around 6,000.

3.46 Turnover of administrative staff was very high as many staff were seconded from other parts of government for short periods of a month or less. Expertise was therefore sometimes lost and, even where there were clear desk instructions, it took time for replacements to get up to speed. New staff from other organisations were understandably unfamiliar with the Department's systems, administrative instructions and lines of accountability, and this created difficulties when they had to carry out contract and financial processing work. Acute shortages of administrative managers meant that inexperienced staff filled many such positions on temporary promotion. In most cases the promoted staff responded well to the challenges of the greater responsibility. From June 2001 onwards problems were also encountered because of a perception by those outside the Department that the fight against the disease had been won. Other government departments and agencies pressed for the return of seconded staff, but these were still needed, particularly on licensing and financial work. These problems occurred throughout the Department both in the field and at headquarters.

Arrangements have been introduced to improve the speed and effectiveness of any future response

3.47 The Department has drawn on its experiences and lessons learned in 2001 and its Interim Contingency Plan of March 2002 includes measures designed to secure a swift and co-ordinated response to any future outbreak of foot and mouth disease. The measures include the prior identification of Regional Operations Directors, along with key administrative, field and specialist staff; and the setting up of a Joint Co-ordination Centre and liaison with the Environment Agency, other Government departments and stakeholders on the first day that an outbreak is confirmed. The Department will also incorporate lessons identified by the Lessons Learned and Royal Society Inquiries into the 2001 outbreak and from working groups it has set up. One of these is considering how best to secure private sector veterinary assistance in the eradication of the disease. Another is considering the benefits of identifying specialist staff who would help to get Disease Control Centres quickly up and running in any future outbreak.

3.48 The Civil Contingencies Secretariat was established within the Cabinet Office in July 2001 and reports to the Prime Minister through the Cabinet Secretary. It was established because the experiences of the fuel protests in 2000, the floods in the winter of 2000 and the outbreak of foot and mouth disease in 2001 highlighted the fact that the Cabinet Office was in the best position to draw together and co-ordinate the different strands of Government activity which come into play in difficult situations, emerge relatively quickly and have implications that go beyond the responsibilities of single departments. Responsibility for the political and strategic direction of any emergency or of any future outbreak of disease would depend on its scale and the resources necessary to deal with it. Decisions on such matters would be taken at the time.

Movement control and biosecurity measures reduced the scale of the 2001 epidemic, but were not always effective in preventing its spread

3.49 The Department's control strategy for stamping out the disease comprised eight main elements **(Figure 31)**. Refinements were introduced as greater understanding was acquired of the nature of the spread of the particular strain of virus responsible and the consequences of particular local circumstances.

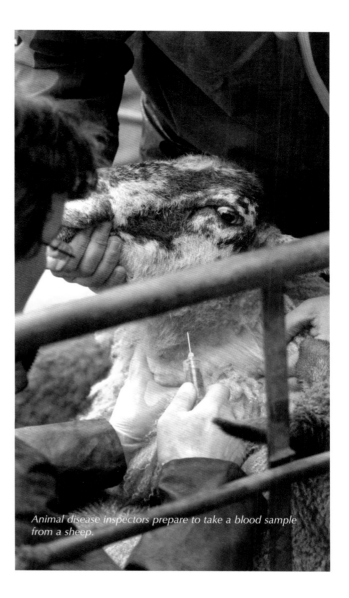

Animal disease inspectors prepare to take a blood sample from a sheep.

---

31   **The main elements of the disease control strategy**

1. Controlling movements of susceptible animals.

2. Maintaining a high level of biosecurity to prevent spread by persons and vehicles that had contact with an infected premises.

3. Rapid reporting, identification and diagnosis of infected animals.

4. Swift tracing of animals which had been exposed to infection.

5. Rapid slaughter of susceptible animals on infected premises or that had been exposed to disease.

   Refinements:

   5 March 2001: Priority given to the slaughter of pigs on infected premises and all susceptible animals on premises contiguous to infected premises with pigs.

   15 March 2001: Slaughter of sheep, goats and pigs on farms within three kilometres of an infected premises in certain parts of Cumbria and Dumfries and Galloway.

   21 March 2001: Slaughter on suspicion of disease of animals that were suspected, on veterinary grounds, to be infected.

   23 March 2001: Target for slaughter of animals on infected premises set at 24 hours of a report of suspicions of the disease; and a new policy to slaughter within 48 hours susceptible animals on premises contiguous to an infected premises. The targets came into effect on 27 March 2001.

   26 April 2001: The 23 March contiguous cull policy refined to enable cattle to escape the cull if they were not clinically infected and there was good biosecurity.

   24 May 2001: Three kilometre cull replaced in Cumbria by serological testing of the sheep flocks.

6. Disposal of carcasses.

7. Preliminary and secondary cleansing and disinfecting of premises.

8. Statistically based serological testing of animals for evidence of current or previous disease to enable restrictions to be lifted safely.

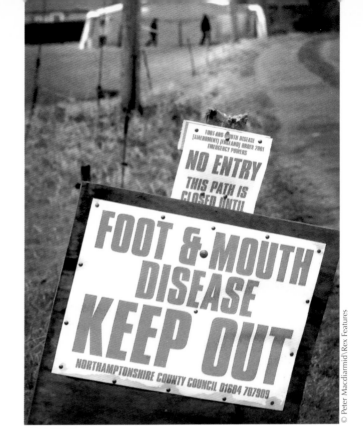

© Peter Macdiarmid\Rex Features

A national movement ban (and closure of livestock markets) on 23 February 2001 prevented greater spread of the disease but with hindsight could have been imposed earlier in this outbreak

3.50 Preventing the movement of infected animals is vital since direct animal to animal contact is the quickest means of virus transmission. On 19 February 2001, in accordance with "Chapter 3" Instructions, the Department imposed a ban on livestock movements in an eight kilometre radius around the first suspect premises (an abattoir in Essex). On 21 February 2001, as required by European Union law and the Foot and Mouth Disease Order 1983, this was extended to 10 kilometres after infection had been confirmed. Movement restrictions were placed around all farms which had been identified as having links with the abattoir. At 5 pm on 23 February 2001, just under three days after confirmation of the first case, a controlled area was established throughout Britain. This involved the closure of livestock markets and a national ban on the movement of susceptible animals. The movement ban was initially imposed temporarily (for seven days) to provide time for tracing livestock "at risk".

3.51 The closure of markets and the national movement standstill were crucial in checking the further spread of the virus to areas where it was not already 'seeded', such as northern Scotland and the pig-based farming areas of central and eastern England. The example of Taiwan, in 1997, where disease spread across the country, affecting four million pigs, as a result of an inability to close pig markets, shows what might have occurred if controls had been more relaxed. In retrospect, it would clearly have been prudent and more effective if the national movement ban had been imposed from the outset. On 20 February 2001, the virus was already 'seeded' in at least nine of the 12 areas of subsequent concentration; and at least 57 farms were infected. Evidence from other outbreaks indicates that a further 20-30 cases per infected farm could be expected. For many weeks the Department was therefore 'chasing' the disease.

3.52 On 20 February 2001 the Department suspended the issue of export certificates for susceptible livestock and on 21 February 2001 the European Union's Standing Veterinary Committee banned related United Kingdom exports. However, the disease spread further over the next few days through livestock markets and movements by dealers. The ban on exports meant that movements were intensified as dealers sought alternative outlets for livestock destined for overseas. By 23 February 2001, a further 62 farms are believed to have become infected. 'Seeding' was intensified in areas already infected and the disease also spread to seven additional counties: Anglesey, Cornwall, Derbyshire, Leicestershire, Oxfordshire, West Yorkshire and Worcestershire. One of the Government's academic advisers has estimated that the overall scale of the outbreak might have been reduced by between a third and a half if a national movement ban had been imposed straightaway on 20 February 2001,[14] although this was based on a developing model and data was subsequently improved.

3.53 The main reason why there was not an immediate countrywide movement ban on 20 February 2001 was that the Department felt that a nationwide ban would not be proportionate. The Department believed that local movement controls would control the disease. A national ban would have been unprecedented and the Department considers that the epidemiological evidence at that time did not exist to justify a countrywide ban. At the early stages of the outbreak the disease was almost exclusively in pigs. The pig industry does not tend to involve multiple nationwide animal movements as occurs in the sheep industry. Even when the national movement ban was introduced, on 23 February 2001, many in the livestock industry criticised it as premature since only five premises, in Essex and Northumberland, had at that time been confirmed with infection.

3.54 In the light of its experience of the 2001 outbreak, the Department announced, in March 2002 in its Interim Contingency Plan, that, were another outbreak to occur, all susceptible animal movements would be stopped countrywide on confirmation of the first case. This approach is supported by a range of bodies who responded to our invitation to comment, for example the Farmers' Union of Wales, the Tenant Farmers Association and the British Meat Federation. The plan is interim and does not seek to pre-judge the outcome of the Lessons Learned and Royal Society Inquiries into the 2001 outbreak.

3.55 To relieve the animal welfare and commercial pressures that can rapidly build up for farmers when normal movements are restricted, the Department allowed licensed movements of animals from early March 2001. Biosecurity and other conditions were attached to the licences.

14 Professor Woolhouse evidence to the Environment, Food and Rural Affairs Select Committee on 7 November 2001.

Because compliance with local control measures was incomplete they were not fully effective in stopping the spread of the disease

3.56 The Department imposed restrictions over the movement of animals, persons and vehicles on and around infected premises, and on the local movements of animals between different parts of an owner's property **(Figure 32)**. These restrictions were supplemented by licensing inspection and biosecurity precautions. Because compliance with these measures was not complete they were not fully effective in preventing the local spread of the disease. From the second week of the outbreak, the disease was chiefly being spread locally over distances of less than three kilometres **(Figure 33)**. Movement of people and vehicles was a significant factor in this local spread. The problems were most acute where farms were not held in compact units, as in parts of Devon and Cumbria, or where owners were accustomed to helping each other perform agricultural tasks, as in the Hexham area of Northumberland.

32 Local movement and biosecurity controls

Statutory controls on and around infected premises

When disease is first suspected, a **Form A** is served on the premises, declaring it to be an **infected place**. No movements are allowed on or off the premises without permission and a disinfectant footbath must be maintained at the entrance.

If after clinical examination the Department's vet suspects that disease is present, a **Form C** is signed. This prohibits the movement of animals within an eight kilometre radius of the premises while laboratory tests results are awaited.

On formal confirmation of the disease, by laboratory test results or on clinical signs, an **Infected Area** is declared, based on a minimum distance of 10 kilometres around the Infected Place, replacing the Form C. Stock movements are banned, livestock vehicles must be thoroughly cleansed and disinfected, and milk can be fed only to animals on the same premises. All premises within a three kilometre protection zone around the infected place are placed under Form D restrictions (see below).

An Infected Area is lifted after clinical examination of cattle and pigs and blood-testing of sheep flocks within the protection zone show no signs of the disease. This cannot happen until at least 30 days have elapsed after preliminary cleansing and disinfecting.

A **Form D** may be imposed on farms, both inside and outside the Infected Area zone, which are believed to have some link to an infected premises. If this link can be classed as a dangerous contact the animals will be killed. Susceptible animals on these farms must be isolated and movement restrictions are imposed on the owner or occupier, who must ensure that anyone leaving the place thoroughly cleanses and disinfects hands, footwear and clothing. These restrictions are for an unlimited period if within the protection zone or for, typically, 21 days if outside, as by then clinical signs of disease would be expected to be apparent during patrols to the premises by Departmental staff.

Licensed local movements

From 9 March 2001, some licensed local movements of animals were allowed outside the most high-risk areas. This included movements between premises in the same ownership and control of up to 10 kilometres, subject to a central check on the premises' disease status and prior veterinary inspection of the animals. Licensed repeat 'occupational movements' of animals across roads on the same holding, for example for milking, were also allowed, without veterinary inspection, initially for welfare reasons but, from late April, also for general management reasons. When crossing roads, owners were expected to ensure that roads were left clean and disinfected.

33 Methods of spread of the disease

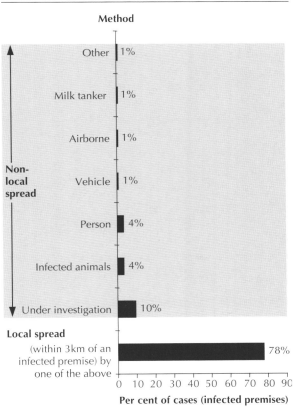

Method

Other 1%

Milk tanker 1%

Airborne 1%

Non-local spread

Vehicle 1%

Person 4%

Infected animals 4%

Under investigation 10%

Local spread (within 3km of an infected premise) by one of the above 78%

0 10 20 30 40 50 60 70 80 90

Per cent of cases (infected premises)

NOTES

1. The Department defined 'local spread' as 'spread between infected premises within three kilometres of each other'.

2. The Department considered that most local spread was attributable either to aerosol spread between animals or from contamination, for example of roads or common facilities, by poor biosecurity on leaving and returning to farms.

Source: The Department's Epidemiology Report of 21 October 2001

3.57 The Department relied on farmers and others to comply with movement and biosecurity controls since they, and local authority trading standards departments[15], had insufficient resources to monitor compliance in depth. A minority did not comply with biosecurity requirements and these breaches contributed to local spread of the disease. In June 2001, a two per cent sample check of local occupational licences by the Department found incomplete compliance with their terms in 30 per cent of licences. However, most infringements were minor and sometimes arose because farmers were confused by conflicting advice about details of disinfecting.

3.58 In only a handful of cases, where there was a wilful breach of the requirement to cleanse and disinfect roads, were matters referred to trading standards for enforcement. By the end of July 2001, local authority trading standards departments were aware also of at least 730 illegal movements, had issued cautions for 195, and were prosecuting in respect of 33. Around a further 30 prosecutions were undertaken in the second half of 2001. By mid-October 2001, there had been more than 30 convictions **(Figure 34)** for unauthorised animal movements, failure to confine animals and other biosecurity breaches. Most involved the movement of only a small number of animals, although only a single infected animal is sufficient to cause the disease to spread. The average fine was £1,000 per case. Farmers found guilty of illegal movements or breaches of biosecurity were still legally entitled to compensation for the slaughter of their animals.

34 Examples of prosecutions for breaches of biosecurity

On 19 March 2001, a Cumbrian farmer allowed fodder to be moved, six days after imposition of movement restrictions on his farm. His livestock were later confirmed as having foot and mouth disease. He was fined £1,000, plus £100 costs.

On 17 April 2001, another Cumbrian farmer moved six sheep locally without a licence. He was fined £250, plus £100 costs.

On 10 May 2001 a North Yorkshire farmer was fined £100 for allowing his animals to stray. He had breached bail conditions that had required him to pen his animals.

NB The maximum that could be imposed for a breach was a fine of £1,000 per animal, up to a maximum of £5,000, and a month's imprisonment.

3.59 There were some breaches of biosecurity by those working with the Department, although the Department considers that the vast majority of those working with it adhered to all biosecurity requirements. The Department told us that any reports of biosecurity breaches by the Department's staff or contractors were taken extremely seriously. When sufficient evidence was provided they were fully investigated. If found to have

any basis appropriate action was taken. Depending on the severity of the breach, this included retraining, removal to other duties and, in some cases, dismissal of the person or contractor. In Exeter, for example, a valuer was suspended for cycling between farms without taking appropriate biosecurity precautions; in Worcester a Temporary Veterinary Inspector was dismissed; and in Newcastle a field officer was reprimanded. Biosecurity protocols were revised to incorporate lessons arising.

3.60 In a small number of cases, vehicles transporting carcasses to rendering plants or mass burial or burn sites developed leaks. The Department told us that these leaks were identified by escort vehicles and appropriate action taken. Some farmers expressed concerns that disease close to the M5 in Cheshire and M6 in Somerset may have been caused by passing rendering vehicles. However, the Department's epidemiologists have investigated these allegations, and also suggestions that veterinary surveillance visits may have spread disease, but have found no epidemiological evidence to support them.

3.61 From the outset, the Department, farmers' unions and other stakeholders collaborated to try to improve farmers' awareness of the importance of biosecurity. The Department sent a biosecurity factsheet to livestock farmers on 5 March 2001 and further advice on 12 and 21 April 2001. The need for greater action was highlighted in May 2001 by the outbreak of a cluster of 20 new cases in Settle, North Yorkshire, 14 of which were associated with movements of people, vehicles or licensed livestock. The Department responded by suspending movement licences in the Settle/Clitheroe area. In early July 2001 the Department also launched an £800,000 publicity campaign. This involved advertising in the regional press and on local radio, Ministerial roadshows and providing a 15 minute biosecurity video to all livestock farmers.

3.62 A further flare-up, around Thirsk in North Yorkshire, led to the imposition, on 29 July 2001, of a 900-square-mile Restricted Infected Area. Vehicles visiting the 2,700 farms within this area had to be licensed and fully cleansed and disinfected before entering and leaving each premises. Staff from the Department accompanied milk tankers, and some grain and feed lorries, to check that they had been disinfected. Staff from local authorities, the police and the Department patrolled the zone 24 hours a day to check on farms, vehicles and the cleanliness of rural lanes. In the Thirsk biosecurity zone, early inspections found that 77 of the 569 vehicles checked were inadequately disinfected; and 80 of the 1,165 farms surveyed lacked footbaths at their entrances. The increased level of monitoring had a positive impact and by mid-September 2001 infringements had fallen to around five per cent of vehicles and footbaths checked, compared with over 15 per cent earlier on.

---

15 Local authority trading standards departments are responsible for a wide range of enforcement activities in respect of animal diseases and animal welfare. During the 2001 outbreak they also had to enforce new rules on animal movements and biosecurity and licence movements of animals to slaughter for human consumption. From September 2001, local authorities were later responsible for issuing most licences under the 'Autumn animal movements' arrangements. The police service also assisted in the enforcement of biosecurity. The Farming and Rural Conservation Agency (now part of the Rural Development Service within the Department) administered the local welfare licence movement scheme until autumn 2001. In Scotland and Wales, the devolved administrations' local agricultural offices issued local movement licences.

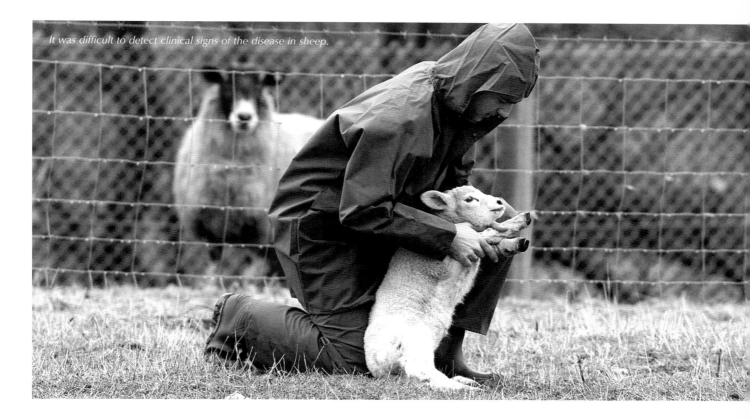

It was difficult to detect clinical signs of the disease in sheep.

3.63 Restricted Infected Areas were also established around Penrith in Cumbria on 7 August 2001; and around Allendale and Hexham in Northumberland on 26 August 2001. These intensified arrangements were important in helping to bring the outbreak to an end. The National Farmers' Union told us that it supported such rigorous measures: they should have been introduced earlier and applied more widely across the country. In March 2002, the Department announced in its Interim Contingency Plan that, subject to the recommendations of the Lessons Learned and Royal Society Inquiries into the 2001 outbreak, the measures would be imposed from day 1 of any future outbreak. The Department emphasises that the use of Restricted Infected Areas as a control measure is resource intensive and requires highly specialised staff from local authorities and the police.

There were difficulties in identifying and diagnosing the disease

3.64 Infected premises were identified in three main ways (**Figure 35**):

- from reports of suspicion of disease by farmers or their private vets (72 per cent of cases);

- during inspection visits by the Department's vets at premises identified as dangerous contacts through information obtained from infected premises (12 per cent of cases); and

- by the Department's vets during patrol visits to inspect livestock on farms in the vicinity of infected premises (10 per cent of cases).

35 **How infected premises were identified**

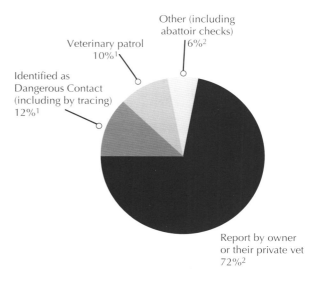

Other (including abattoir checks) 6%[2]

Veterinary patrol 10%[1]

Identified as Dangerous Contact (including by tracing) 12%[1]

Report by owner or their private vet 72%[2]

NOTES

1. By the Department.
2. By others.

Source: National Audit Office analysis of data in the Department's Disease Control System.

There were difficulties in detecting the clinical signs of disease

3.65 Farmers and their private vets are required to report any suspicions of infection promptly. Prompt reporting was necessary if the Department were to act quickly to check the spread of the disease. However, reporting was slower in 2001 than in 1967-68 and this contributed to the scale of the outbreak. In 1967-68 most cases of the disease were only one day old at the time of report. In 2001 diseased cattle were typically diagnosed two days after clinical signs and sheep five days or more after clinical signs. These delays arose in part from a reduced awareness of foot and mouth disease among farmers and private vets, but mainly because sheep were the main species affected in 2001 whereas the 1967-68 outbreak was cattle-based. The disease is much more difficult to detect in sheep than in cattle and pigs: sheep display clinical signs only for a short period of time; and the disease spreads slowly through a flock with only a few individuals showing clinical signs at any one time. In the 2001 outbreak, visible lesions were often found in only a small percentage of sheep in infected flocks. The 2001 virus strain also produced signs similar to those of other ovine diseases.

3.66 The Department provided farmers with illustrated factsheets of clinical signs to look for and what to do if they had any suspicions of foot and mouth disease in their animals. Nevertheless, the difficulties in identification meant that some outbreaks were reported late, as illustrated by the outbreak in Settle in May 2001 (**Figure 36**), or were not reported at all. In addition, many false reports were made. The Department encouraged reporting in the knowledge that many reports would be false alarms. Three-quarters of farmers' reports were false alarms and two-thirds of early suspected cases sent to the Institute for Animal Health's laboratory tested negative for the disease.

The Department faced resource and operational constraints in identification and diagnosis

3.67 The Department was faced early on with a massive veterinary and administrative workload. It had to trace the movement of more than 100,000 sheep through potentially infected livestock markets during the weeks before 23 February 2001; visit farms where disease was suspected; and regularly patrol farms in the zones surrounding infected premises. Tracing work was hampered by a failure of some farmers to keep movement records; by some unrecorded transactions occurring outside official markets; and by there being no requirement for individual identification of sheep.[16] On 8 March 2001 the Department publicly sought help from farmers and dealers in tracing movements outside official markets.

3.68 The Department had planned to carry out surveillance patrols of livestock every 48 hours within the three kilometre protection zone around infected premises. The scale of the requirement was enormous: as early as 20 March 2001 it was calculated that some 8,365 premises would have to be visited within the protection zones. Shortages of available vets meant that these patrols had to be scaled back in many areas and were abandoned altogether in Cumbria. These premises were nevertheless under restrictions and the farmers were required to report any suspicion of disease.

3.69 In "clean areas" with no identified link with infected animals, premises would be confirmed as infected once a positive laboratory result had been obtained from samples sent to the Institute for Animal Health's laboratory at Pirbright. This posed a huge logistical challenge for the Institute as its Pirbright laboratory typically tested around 500 field samples for vesicular disease virus analysis a year. In week 2 of the outbreak it had to deal with diagnostic (virological) samples from 161 premises where disease was suspected: for each

---

36 **The Settle outbreak in May 2001 - an illustration of the difficulties of identifying foot and mouth disease in sheep**

A local outbreak of 55 infected premises in the Settle area of North Yorkshire between 10 May and 16 July 2001 presented the most striking example of difficulties in identifying infection in sheep during the 2001 epidemic and the consequences in an area with mixed (sheep and cattle) family-run farms.

On 19 February 2001, infection was introduced inadvertently into the area by the truck of a livestock haulier who had transported sheep from Longtown market, in Cumbria, on 15 February 2001. Disease circulated, undetected, among sheep on the farm that had been visited by the livestock haulier and only became apparent, in early May 2001, when cattle were infected. This occurred in April 2001, after they were turned out from indoor sheds to graze in fields where sheep had also grazed.

Farming in the Settle area was characterised by extensive family-run units of dairy cattle, beef cattle and sheep. Many farms had parcels of land away from the home premises. Consequently, there were considerable movements of farm personnel, feed lorries and milk tankers between premises, as well as several hundred licensed local animal movements. These movements, along with, in the Department's judgement, poor biosecurity on some farms, contributed to local dissemination of the disease.

Source: National Audit Office analysis of the Department's epidemiological reports.

---

16 *Cattle have unique ear tag numbers and 'passports' and their movement is tracked on the computerised Cattle Tracing System run by the British Cattle Movement Service, which is part of the Department and is based in Workington. Pigs are not identified individually, but are controlled in batches and must be accompanied by a movement licence when leaving a premises. There is no individual identification system for sheep though sheep movements must be recorded.*

premises, an average of around five samples were received. By week 12 its workload had risen to a peak of 289 such cases and over the course of the epidemic, between 19 February and 30 September 2001, it received 15,400 diagnostic samples from the United Kingdom . The Institute responded well, quadrupling the staffing of its testing section to provide a seven days a week, 24 hours a day service. Turnaround times averaged 26 hours during weeks 1-3 of the epidemic. They were as fast as 3-4 hours when the initial antigen test gave a positive result. Where the antigen test result was negative, up to two passages in tissue culture were needed, taking up to four days to confirm a negative result.

The Department made a number of changes to get round these constraints

3.70 In mid-March 2001 the Government was presented with evidence from its scientific advisers that because the Department was initially having to "chase" the disease this could potentially lead to an exponential growth in the number of new cases. This reflected the widespread seeding of the disease in February 2001 before the first case had been identified. On 12 March 2001, the Department's Epidemiological Modelling Team advised that around two-thirds of infected premises might be unidentified at any time and that "current control measures are insufficient to control the epidemic".

3.71 On 13 March 2001 epidemiological researchers at Imperial College, Edinburgh University and Cambridge University were sent the Department's disease control data, and regular updates from that point onwards. On 16 March 2001, epidemiological research groups from Imperial College and Edinburgh University supplied separate preliminary analyses to the Chief Veterinary Officer which indicated that current control measures were insufficient to control the epidemic. On 21 March 2001 epidemiologists warned that the epidemic would continue to grow exponentially if control measures in place in mid-March were not intensified. Their initial worst-case scenario suggested approximately 1,000 cases per day might occur by mid-May if the control measures in place in mid-March were not changed. It was proposed that rapid slaughter of animals at infected farms and surrounding farms within 1.5 kilometres of infected farms would be sufficient to control the epidemic, reducing the scale by two-thirds. This proposal was put to a meeting held in the Cabinet Office on 22 March 2001. As a result of model refinements and more data from the Department the worst-case figure was scaled back to approximately 400 cases a day in projections made on 29 March 2001 **(Figure 37 overleaf)**[17]. This information was presented to the Cabinet Office Briefing Room on 30 March 2001.

3.72 As soon as the nature of the outbreak was recognised the Department responded by introducing a number of changes in approach:

- On 15 March 2001, the Minister of Agriculture announced that, to speed up diagnosis, the disease was being confirmed on the basis of vets' clinical diagnoses. In fact confirmation on clinical grounds before laboratory tests results were received had been taking place in many cases from as early as 21 February 2001.

- On 15 March 2001, the Department approved a cull of 700,000 sheep on 2,000 premises in north Cumbria and southwest Scotland which lay within three kilometres of infected premises and were considered to have been exposed to the risk of infection by 'seeding' from Longtown market. The cull began on 22 March 2001 and ended in mid-May.

- From 21 March 2001, the Department allowed the "slaughter on suspicion" of all susceptible animals on a premises where a vet suspected infection but there was insufficient clinical and epidemiological evidence to be certain it was foot and mouth disease.

- On 23 March 2001, based on the analyses presented by the Chief Scientific Adviser from the modellers, the decision was made to slaughter susceptible animals on premises contiguous to infected premises. Contiguous premises were those in the neighbourhood of infected premises where it was believed that animals had been exposed to infection. This decision was informed by analyses, carried out separately by the Department's Epidemiological Modelling Team and researchers at Imperial College and Cambridge University, which showed that farms within 1.5 kilometres of infected premises had a 17 per cent chance of later being infected. The Imperial Team advised that it was too risky to wait for infection to be identified during patrol visits: cases would inevitably be missed. This judgement was supported by other epidemiologists. They recommended prompt contiguous culling to reduce the scale of the epidemic dramatically. The Department's Epidemiological Modelling Team also advised that the slaughter of animals on contiguous premises, and quicker identification and slaughter at infected premises, might help to halve the overall size of the epidemic, which they predicted could reach 4,000 cases[18]. The targets of 24 hours to cull animals at infected premises and 48 hours to cull animals at contiguous premises were set at this time.

17 The foot and mouth epidemic in Great Britain: pattern of spread and impact of interventions, N M Ferguson, C A Donnelly, R M Anderson (Science 2001 Vol 292 pp 1155 - 1160, published on line 12 April 2001)
18 Predictive spatial modelling of alternative control strategies for the foot-and-mouth disease epidemic in Great Britain, 2001, RS Morris, JW Wilesmith, MW Stern, RL Sanson, MA Stevenson (The Veterinary Record, 4 August 2001, pp. 137-43).

37 **The Imperial College team's epidemiological model predictions of 29 March 2001 and a comparison with the actual path of the epidemic**

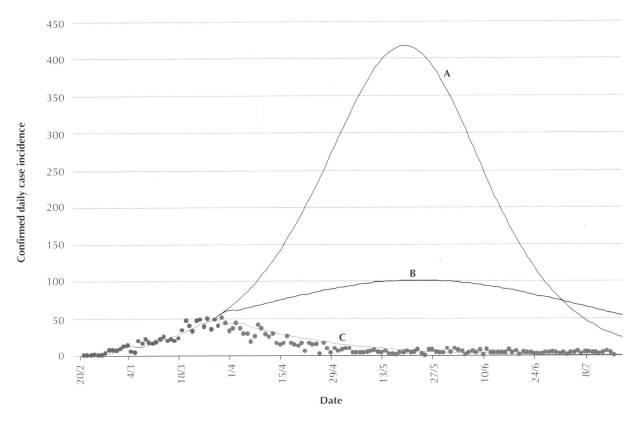

A: Several days to slaughter

B: Slaughter on infected premises

C: Slaughter on infected and neighbouring farms within 24 and 48 hours, respectively

● Data up to 29 March

● Data from 30 March

NOTE

The Imperial College team predicted that around three-quarters of farms in affected areas would be infected and culled if there was no change in strategy or performance (line A) as compared to a fifth if the 24hrs/48hrs slaughter strategy was implemented and achieved (line C).

Source: Imperial College

These changes helped to control the disease but led to the culling of many animals which may have been exposed but were not showing clinical signs of the disease

3.73 The intensified culling strategy, along with other disease control measures, such as restrictions on livestock movements, helped to check the growth in new confirmed cases, which peaked on 30 March 2001. Thereafter, the decline was similar to, but initially sharper than, that predicted by the Imperial Team's model. The Government's Chief Scientific Adviser told the Select Committee on Environment, Food and Rural Affairs on 7 November 2001 that the contiguous cull policy, although not carried out perfectly, had helped to bring the disease under control.

3.74 **Figure 38** shows the results of laboratory tests on animals culled on the basis of vets' clinical diagnoses, on animals slaughtered on suspicion of having the disease and on animals slaughtered because they were in dangerous contact with infected premises or as part of the contiguous cull.

3.75 Where slaughter was based on clinical diagnoses, samples were taken in many cases and sent for laboratory analysis. Some 78 per cent of these tests were positive suggesting that veterinary diagnoses were correct in more than three-quarters of cases. Veterinary diagnoses not confirmed by a laboratory may have occurred:

■ because a negative laboratory test does not necessarily mean that the disease was not present as the animal tested could have been in the process of incubating the disease[19].

■ because of the inherent difficulties of diagnosing the disease in sheep; and

■ because of the inexperience of some temporary veterinary inspectors, some of whom were recently qualified or did not specialise in farm livestock, although in many cases there was the opportunity for a second veterinary opinion to be sought.

38 **The proportion of premises in which laboratory tests gave a positive result for the presence of the foot and mouth disease virus**

	Infected premises confirmed on clinical grounds[1]	Slaughter on Suspicion cases[2]	Contiguous premises classified as dangerous contacts	Other Dangerous Contact cases
Tested positive	78 per cent	16 per cent	30 per cent (see warning note)	41 per cent (see warning note)
Tested negative	22 per cent	84 per cent (see warning note)	70 per cent (see warning note)	59 per cent (see warning note)
Proportion of cases for which samples were taken and results are available.	90 per cent	78 per cent	5 per cent	8 per cent
Number of animals slaughtered[3]	1.1 million	0.1 million	1.2 million	8 per cent

WARNING NOTE

These figures are not based on random samples and should not be taken as representative of the population of contiguous or dangerous contact cases as a whole. The figures for the percentages which tested positive are likely to overstate the overall rate of infection in contiguous and dangerous contact premises since many of the cases tested would be for animals showing clinical signs of disease for which the test results would be expected to be positive.

OTHER NOTES

1. Over the course of the epidemic, nine-tenths of infected premises were confirmed on clinical grounds. The results shown here exclude infected premises that originated as dangerous contact or slaughter on suspicion cases. If these are included, the proportion tested as positive would fall to 74 per cent.

2. Results include those cases which originated as slaughter on suspicion or dangerous contact premises, but which were later classed as infected premises, on the basis of laboratory results or clinical evidence.

3. The figures exclude many slaughtered new born lambs and calves who were not counted in the Department's database because their value, for compensation purposes, was included in the valuation assigned to their mother.

Source: The Department

19 *Some negative laboratory results may have been 'false negatives', arising from damage to the sample in transit or from animals being in the process of incubating the disease. Moreover, on suspected infected premises vets took samples from only a relatively small number of animals they considered most likely to be infected. In the case of sheep flocks, this meant that samples may not have been taken from some infected animals.*

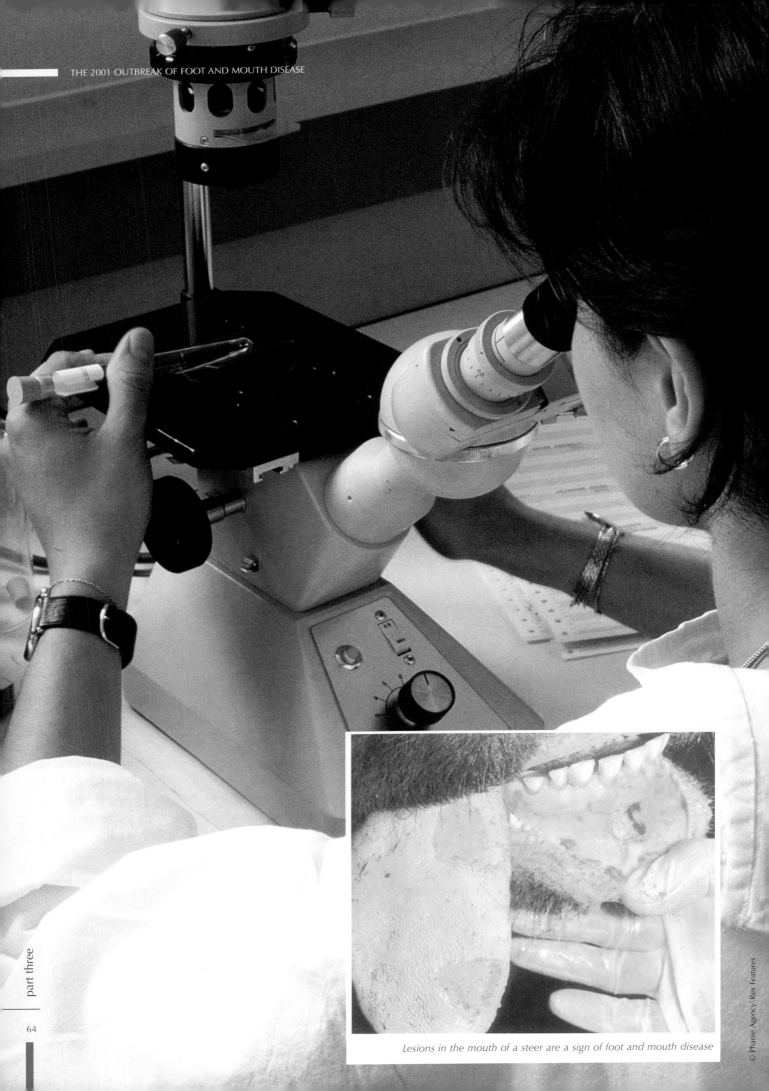

Lesions in the mouth of a steer are a sign of foot and mouth disease

3.76 There were considerable differences across Disease Control Centres in the proportion of positive laboratory test results for infected premises, ranging from highs of 90 to 95 per cent in Carlisle, Chelmsford and Leeds to lows of 30 to 50 per cent for Gloucester, Worcester, Stafford and Caernarfon. In the latter four Disease Control Centres, there were not positive test results for the disease in 150 of the 247 "confirmed infected" premises, though, for the reasons stated above, this does not necessarily mean that disease was not present. In certain disease clusters, for example, in the Black Mountains area of Wales, with seven infected premises, and the Builth Wells and Cardiff-Newport clusters, each with three infected premises, none of the clinical diagnoses were backed up by positive laboratory test results. However, this does not mean that the disease was not present in these areas. In the Black Mountains, for example, specimens were not submitted for sampling from the infected premises where there was the most convincing clinical evidence.

3.77 Where slaughter was based on suspicion of the disease, laboratory tests were undertaken in most cases: 16 per cent of these cases tested positive. Where slaughter was based on dangerous contacts or was part of the contiguous cull, laboratory tests were also undertaken, although in only a small number of cases. Some 30 per cent of contiguous premises and 41 per cent of other dangerous contact premises tested positive. These figures must be treated with caution, however. They are not based on random samples and should not be taken as representative of the population of contiguous or dangerous contact cases as a whole. The figures are likely to overstate the overall rate of infection since many of the cases tested would be for animals showing clinical signs of disease for which the test results would be expected to be positive.

3.78 The contiguous cull strategy was based on the understanding that, whilst there would inevitably be some slaughter of animals not showing clinical signs of disease from disease-free premises, the strategy would remove animals incubating the disease, enable quicker eradication and reduce the overall number of infected animals and premises. Some vets and scientists argued that there had been unnecessary rigidity in its application. They believed that there should have been more room for local judgement, informed by such factors as topography and assessed risks of exposure. Throughout, the veterinary assessment to determine whether it was necessary to carry out slaughter on individual contiguous premises had to be against a background that susceptible animals were believed to have been exposed to disease and in accordance with the Animal Health Act 1981, which provides for exceptions to slaughter to be granted on the basis of local veterinary judgement. One of the Department's expert advisers, Dr Alex Donaldson of the Institute for Animal Health (a member of the Foot and Mouth Disease Science Group), considered[20] that "The action taken on contiguous premises should therefore be determined by the species at risk on those premises. In the case of sheep, which may have been exposed to an infectious plume of virus, culling would be justified since foot and mouth disease in that species is often mild or inapparent and so clinical surveillance would be of limited value in determining whether a flock was infected or not. For cattle, intensified clinical surveillance would be an appropriate alternative to immediate culling, since foot and mouth disease in that species is easily recognised and any cases should be quickly identified and eliminated before there was a risk of infectious plumes of virus being generated."

3.79 From 26 April 2001, with more veterinary resources now available for patrolling, the Department allowed case-by-case local veterinary risk assessment where cattle and certain rare sheep breeds were involved. This involved veterinary consideration of the risk of exposure and adequacy of biosecurity. In Wales, there had been local veterinary risk assessment from the outset, at the insistence of the Welsh Assembly's Rural Affairs Minister. The National Farmers' Union accepted the necessity of the contiguous and three-kilometre culls, but welcomed the greater flexibility that was introduced at a later stage to allow more targeted culling of dangerous contacts on contiguous farms according to vets' judgements of the adequacy of biosecurity on neighbouring farms.

3.80 Neither the contiguous cull nor, in north Cumbria, the three kilometre cull were carried out fully. Slaughter did not take place on a seventh of designated contiguous farms. In Devon around a fifth of affected farmers requested the Disease Control Centre to review its decision to cull. The Department decided not to proceed in some cases where it was considered that, although parts of a farm were contiguous to an infected premises, the area where livestock was kept was not, and biosecurity was effective. Opposition was fiercest from owners of prime cattle and 'hobby farmers', who kept small numbers of livestock to supplement other income. On 24 April 2001, Exeter's Regional Operations Director advised the Department that the policy "was increasingly being seen not to be capable of application". In Dumfries and Galloway the three kilometre and contiguous culls were implemented more fully and helped quickly to confine the outbreak. Elsewhere, the cattle and rare breeds exemptions announced on 26 April 2001 aimed to address farmers' concerns.

---

20 A I Donaldson, S Alexandersen, J H Sorensen and T Mikkelsen, 'Relative risks of the uncontrollable (airborne) spread of foot and mouth disease by different species' (Veterinary Record, 12 May 2001, pp 603-604).

3.81 The contiguous cull was hugely controversial. The Select Committee on Environment, Food and Rural Affairs commented on the "vast and understandable anguish" caused by the relentless slaughter of animals as a result of the contiguous cull policy. The Report of the Public Inquiry set up by Northumberland County Council considered that the policy "may have led in Northumberland to the slaughter of substantially more animals than was needed to contain and eradicate the disease". Evidence presented to the Devon Foot and Mouth Inquiry was "overwhelmingly critical of the balance of effective need against unnecessary killing of healthy stock under the contiguous cull policy". On the basis of the advice from its veterinary and scientific advisers, however, the Department considers that at the time the contiguous cull was the only way to bring the disease under control. The Department believes that it saved many animal lives by containing the spread of the disease.

The Department was unable in some cases to achieve the rapid slaughter of infected or exposed animals

Performance was worse before new targets for infected and contiguous premises came into force on 27 March 2001

3.82 To prevent further spread of the disease, animals identified as being infected or exposed needed to be slaughtered quickly. Slaughter speeds were slower in 2001 than in 1967-68, when more than 70 per cent of animals were culled on infected and "dangerous contact" farms within 24 hours of diagnosis and only two per cent after more than 48 hours. However, livestock densities were higher in 2001 than in 1967-68 and sheep were the main species affected. Farms were also smaller in 1967-68 making gathering and handling of animals for examination and slaughter more straightforward and quicker. On average three times more animals needed to be culled on each infected premises in 2001 compared with 1967-68 and it took more time to gather the animals together. The contiguous and three kilometre culls were also new factors in 2001. Overall 10 times the number of animals were slaughtered for disease control purposes in 2001 than in the 1967-68 outbreak.

3.83 During the first five weeks of the 2001 epidemic, the time taken from report to slaughter[21] was more than 48 hours for over half of infected premises (**Figures 39 opposite and Figure 40 on page 68**). For dangerous contact premises, the interval between identification and slaughter[22] was over 72 hours on four-fifths of premises, with slaughter typically taking between five

and seven days (**Figures 39 and Figure 41 on page 69**). Veterinary instructions required that the slaughter of clinically affected animals should take place immediately and the slaughter of others should be achieved "with all practical speed", although no formal targets were in place at the time. Where slaughter was delayed, compliance with the other measures in place as a result of the restriction notice served would reduce the risks of further disease spread.

3.84 The three main factors contributing to delays in slaughter were:

- **Shortages of resources**: vets, valuers, slaughtermen and equipment. Vets were the key constraint, delaying the speed of response to farmers' reports. On occasion, delays in obtaining the valuer requested by the farmer added a day or more to the time to slaughter. Some items of equipment, such as captive bolt guns, broke down because of overuse and had to be replaced.

- **Inspection and diagnosis protocols**: Occasional delays may have occurred when laboratory results for the initial antigen test were inconclusive. There was also initially a requirement that during a report visit the Department's vet should check *all* livestock before carrying out a detailed clinical examination of the affected animal(s). In addition, at the beginning of the outbreak, vets were not permitted to undertake another visit within five days of visiting an infected premises. This constraint was addressed on 10 March 2001 (see paragraph 3.42).

- **Logistical factors**: the time needed to round up large flocks of sheep and inefficient early arrangements to ensure the co-ordinated arrival of valuers, slaughtermen and disposal teams.

Performance improved from late March 2001 onwards

3.85 On 23 March 2001, a target was announced for slaughter on infected premises within 24 hours of a farmer's report. The Department's vets were expected to arrive at premises within two hours of the report. Slaughter was prioritised by species, in the descending order of pigs, cattle and sheep, to reflect relative transmission risks. A target was also set for the culling of susceptible animals on farms contiguous to infected premises within 48 hours of confirmation of infection. Both targets were communicated to Disease Control Centres on 26 March 2001. Veterinary and scientific advice was that the 24-hour target for infected premises was particularly critical for disease control.

3.86 Slaughter speeds improved, particularly on infected premises, with the discipline of targets in place. From mid-April 2001 the 24-hour report to slaughter target

---

21 *The time taken from a farmer's report of suspicions of the disease to the last susceptible animal on the premises being slaughtered.*
22 *The time taken from the report of disease on the infected premises that gives rise to the dangerous contact to the last susceptible animal on the dangerous contact premises being slaughtered.*

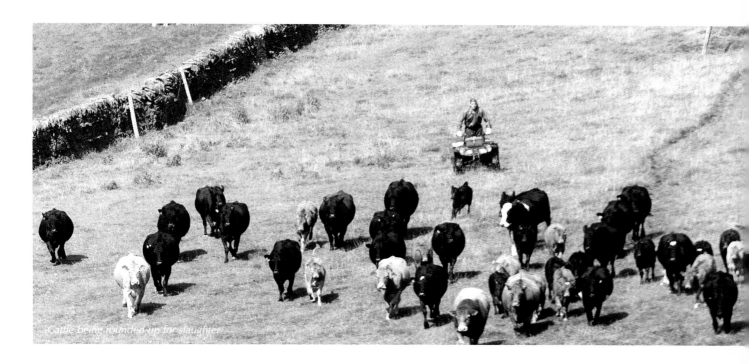

Cattle being rounded up for slaughter

39 Time to slaughter performance

Infected premises (note 1)	Number of premises analysed (note 2)	Within 24 hours %	>24 to 36 hours %	>36 to 48 hours %	More than 48 hours %
Pre 27 March 2001	424	14	24	10	52
Post 27 March 2001	1,101	51	35	4	10
Over entire epidemic	**1.525**	**41**	**32**	**6**	**22**

Premises classified as dangerous contacts and contiguous to an infected premises (note 3)	Number of premises analysed (note 2)	Within 24 hours %	>24 to 48 hours %	>48 to 72 hours %	More than 72 hours %
Pre 27 March 2001	452	1	5	6	88
Post 27 March 2001	2,697	11	34	18	37
Over entire epidemic	**3,149**	**9**	**30**	**17**	**44**

Other dangerous contact premises (notes 3 and 4)	Number of premises analysed (note 2)	Within 24 hours %	>24 to 48 hours %	>48 to 72 hours %	More than 72 hours %
Pre 27 March 2001	866	5	10	10	75
Post 27 March 2001	2,054	10	18	12	60
Over entire epidemic	**2,920**	**9**	**15**	**11**	**65**

NOTES

1. The time taken from a farmer's report of suspicions of the disease to the last susceptible animal on the infected premises being slaughtered. The analysis excludes infected premises that had originated as dangerous contacts or slaughter on suspicion cases.

2. Certain premises could not be analysed because of incompleteness in the available data on times of report and/or slaughter.

3. The time taken from the confirmation of disease on the infected premises that gives rise to the dangerous contact to the last susceptible animal on the dangerous contact premises being slaughtered.

4. At no point during the epidemic were time to slaughter targets in place for dangerous contact premises.

Source: National Audit Office analysis of the data in the Department's Disease Control System.

part three

40   **Report to slaughter times for infected premises during the 2001 outbreak**

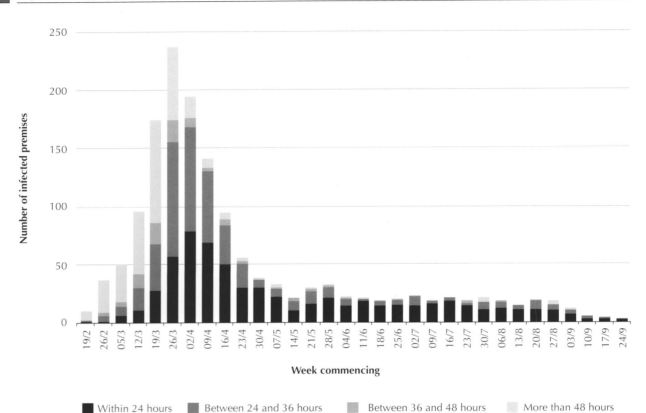

Week commencing

■ Within 24 hours   ■ Between 24 and 36 hours   ■ Between 36 and 48 hours   ■ More than 48 hours

NOTE

The elapsed times shown are those between the report of suspicions of disease and the slaughter of the last susceptible animal.

Source: National Audit Office analysis of the records of 1,525 infected premises for which clear information was available on report and slaughter times. The data was extracted from the Department's Disease Control System.

was achieved on more than half of infected premises. On less than a tenth of premises did slaughter take more than 36 hours. The key changes that secured this improvement were:

■ an increase in veterinary and other resources; and

■ improvements in logistical arrangements, with the formation of dedicated 'infected premises cells' and allocation systems that enabled vets to move quickly on to new premises after organising the slaughter arrangements.

3.87 For 'dangerous contact' premises, slaughter speeds also improved from 26 March 2001, though the change was less dramatic. By late April 2001, slaughter within 48 hours was being achieved on around a half of 'dangerous contact' premises and within 72 hours on around three-quarters. The improvement was less marked than for infected premises because:

■ **The identification of relevant premises took time**: Geographical Information Systems technology proved invaluable during the crisis to produce maps of adjacent premises. However, land ownership and attached parcels of land were sometimes difficult to identify, and not all livestock owners had registered with the Department as they are legally required to do and so were not on its database. This meant that some premises had to be identified through patrols and visits. Owners also had to be contacted and informed.

■ **Some farmers challenged the contiguous cull**: This took the form, on occasions, of refusing access to premises, which sometimes forced the Department to take out a High Court injunction. More commonly, farmers formally requested the Department to reconsider its decision to cull while there were also some challenges in court.

41 **Elapsed time to slaughter for dangerous contact premises during the 2001 outbreak**

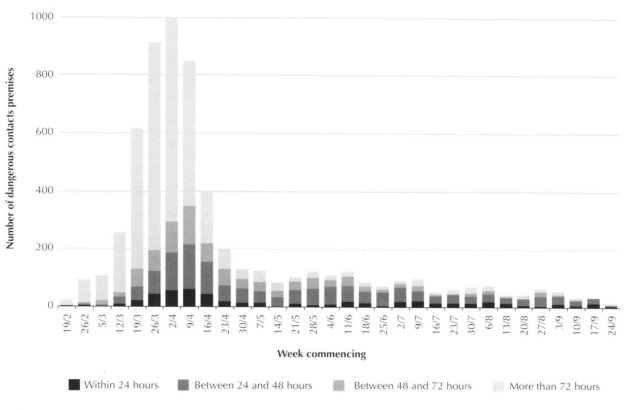

Week commencing

■ Within 24 hours   ■ Between 24 and 48 hours   ■ Between 48 and 72 hours   ■ More than 72 hours

NOTE

The elapsed times shown are those between the confirmation of disease on the related infected premises and slaughter of the last susceptible animal on the dangerous contact premises.

Source: National Audit Office analysis of the records of 6,069 dangerous contact premises for which clear information was available on time to slaughter. The data was extracted from the Department's Disease Control System.

- **The scale and logistics were immense**: Each infected premises was typically surrounded by as many as six contiguous premises, substantially increasing the number of animals that had to be slaughtered and disposed of. In some areas the farming practices meant that premises could be surrounded by stock on several dozen parcels of land, the owners of each of which required tracing.

3.88 The speed with which slaughter was necessary to control the disease and its impact on animal welfare raised concerns from a number of animal welfare organisations (**Figure 42 overleaf**).

Some scientists consider that local spread of the disease would have been reduced if slaughter targets had been met more fully

3.89 Epidemiological analyses have shown that the outbreak would have been considerably larger in scale if extra resources had not been provided in March and April 2001 to reduce the time from reporting to slaughter. They also suggest that a consequence of the failure to reach culling speed targets was to increase local spread of the disease. The Imperial College team calculated that if the '24 hours/48 hours' policy had been fully implemented from 1 April 2001 and the time targets met the number of infected premises would probably have been 16 per cent fewer and the number of farms culled would have been 30 per cent less.[23] This would have meant that more than a million animals would have been spared.

23 *Transmission intensity and the impact of control policies on the foot and mouth epidemic in Great Britain, N M Ferguson, C A Donnelly, R M Anderson (Nature, 4 October 2001, Vol 413, pp 542-548).*

42 Speed of slaughter and its impact on animal welfare

'A balance must be struck between disease control and welfare but welfare must not be set aside even in an emergency'
Farm Animal Welfare Council, 2002

The setting of an explicit target for speed of slaughter, with daily performance reported on the Department's website, posed risks that slaughter standards might be compromised. Furthermore, slaughtermen were paid on a piece rate, rather than hourly, basis. This type of incentive was criticised by the Farm Animal Welfare Council as 'not consistent with welfare-friendly handling and accuracy'. The Royal Society for the Prevention of Cruelty to Animals (RSPCA), in their submission to us, were also critical. They noted that, "where teams were paid on a daily rate, such as at the Great Orton (Cumbria) site, RSPCA staff observed orderly, sensitive and efficient slaughter. Conversely, a piece rate meant that relatively large sums of money could be earned by cutting corners ... (so that) poor slaughter procedures were reportedly relatively common."

The key controls to ensure humane slaughter in accordance with the Welfare of Animals (Slaughter or Killing) Regulations 1995 were: the use only of licensed slaughtermen and audit of the slaughter arrangements by the Department's vets, who were also responsible for killing, by lethal injection, young lambs and calves. Observers from the RSPCA and the Humane Slaughter Association were also on hand at some culls. The Department informed us that slaughter was supervised by qualified veterinary inspectors who were responsible for and took action to maintain standards of welfare at slaughter. Such action included re-training and providing further supervision to slaughtermen and, if necessary, terminating contracts with immediate effect.

The RSPCA told us that they had 'grave concern' at the level of supervision by the Department's vets as a result of resources being stretched. 'In some cases one temporary veterinary inspector could be charged with supervising up to 10 slaughter sites simultaneously'. They were also critical of the length of time taken by the Department to issue clear instructions to staff about the need to pith animals which had been stunned to destroy brain tissue fully. 'This led to a significant number of animals regaining consciousness after stunning, causing great suffering'.

The RSPCA and Compassion in World Farming told us that they had received many reports of improper slaughter methods. The RSPCA investigated over 90 such cases, of which more than 20 required detailed investigation. It appeared to the RSPCA's investigating officers that in many cases there was very good circumstantial evidence that an offence had been committed but, without physical evidence, since the carcasses had been disposed of, prosecution would be fruitless.

3.90 Other modellers have calculated that if the '24 hours/48 hours' strategy had been in place from day 1 and had been fully achieved the overall number of infected premises and animals slaughtered could have been reduced by 40 per cent.[24] It is not realistic, however, to expect to have everything fully operational on day 1 as this would require maintaining vets, other staff and resources at levels that would be impossible to justify in the absence of an outbreak on the scale of that in 2001.

3.91 The Department's epidemiologists have also been researching the course of the epidemic with a view to understanding the impact of control measures. For example, they have carried out some research which involved comparing the dates on which the disease was confirmed with estimated dates of infection. The epidemiologists found that although the peak of the epidemic curve according to the confirmation date was in the week beginning 29 March 2001, the peak of the infection curve was 11 days earlier. They suggest that the peak of infection was at approximately the same time that standard control measures started to have a beneficial effect at the national level as the Department had now "caught up" with the disease. The continued fall in the incidence of infection thereafter was due to a combination of factors including the existing measures, the contiguous cull of animals exposed to infection and an increase in resources including logistical expertise provided by the armed services.

3.92 The Chief Scientific Adviser considers that the contiguous cull was an essential factor in the control of the disease. In a paper on the contiguous cull presented to the Lessons Learned and Royal Society Inquiries, he points out that infections which had already occurred would not have been reported as infected if the farms were removed by the contiguous cull. He considers that this resulted in an immediate drop in the incidence of reported cases when contiguous culling was introduced and that implementation of the contiguous cull also had an immediate effect on the curves of estimated date of infection against time. The turning point on that curve is therefore close to the date on which the contiguous cull was first being effectively implemented. The Chief Scientific Adviser considers that, when these factors are properly taken into account, the timings of the observed peaks in the incidence of estimated new infections or of newly reported cases are both entirely consistent with a significant impact of the contiguous cull on the transmission of foot and mouth disease.

3.93 The Chief Scientific Adviser considers that this effect can also be explained in a way which does not rely on modelling. If animals on a contiguous premises were incubating the disease on, say, 28 March 2001 and were not culled, as was the policy prior to 24 March 2001, they would go on to develop symptoms on, say, 30 March 2001 and would be assigned a date of infection, say 25 March 2001; these cases would appear on the estimated infection date curve and be assigned to 25 March 2001. But if they were culled as a contiguous premises on 28 March 2001, they would not contribute to the cases counted as having been infected on 25 March 2001, because they would not have been showing symptoms on the date of culling. Subsequent serological tests on the culled animals are unlikely to

---

24 *Dynamics of the 2001 UK Foot and Mouth Disease Epidemic: Stochastic Dispersal in a Heterogenous Landscape, M J Keeling, M E J Woolhouse, D J Shaw, L Matthews, M Chase-Topping, D T Haydon, S J Cornell, K Kappey, J Wilesmith, B T Grenfell (Science Express, 4 October 2001, Table 1, p 7).*

pick up antibodies at this stage. The implementation of the contiguous cull policy on a given date would therefore begin to affect the plot of date-of-infection against time at an earlier date.

3.94 The '24 hours/48 hours' slaughter targets are a key element of the Department's Interim Contingency Plan for dealing with any future outbreaks of foot and mouth disease. The policy assumption is for susceptible animals at infected premises to be culled within 24 hours of the disease being reported and all dangerous contacts to be traced and dealt with within a target of 48 hours. Subject to veterinary judgement, contiguous premises will also have a 48 hours to slaughter target. The Department told us that these and other aspects of its Interim Contingency Plan will be revisited in the light of the recommendations of the Lessons Learned and Royal Society Inquiries.

There was a backlog in disposing of slaughtered animals

3.95 Rapid disposal of carcasses is not critical to disease control, unless it holds up slaughter. The risk of disease transmission from carcasses is low as the virus is not produced after the animal is killed. The risk is reduced by regular disinfecting and PVC covering of the heads and feet of infected animals and the restrictions in place at affected premises. After 30 days or so, natural decomposition destroys the virus. However, carcasses awaiting disposal are at risk of attack from scavengers, which theoretically may spread the disease, though in this outbreak no spread by this route has been confirmed. They are also a distressing sight for farmers and the public.

3.96 The sheer scale of the epidemic made disposal a critical problem during 2001. On infected premises, disposal speeds were particularly slow until the third week of April 2001 when, for the first time, disposal was completed on more than half of infected premises within 24 hours of slaughter (**Figure 43**). Until then, the daily

---

43 Elapsed time between completion of slaughter and disposal for infected premises during the 2001 outbreak

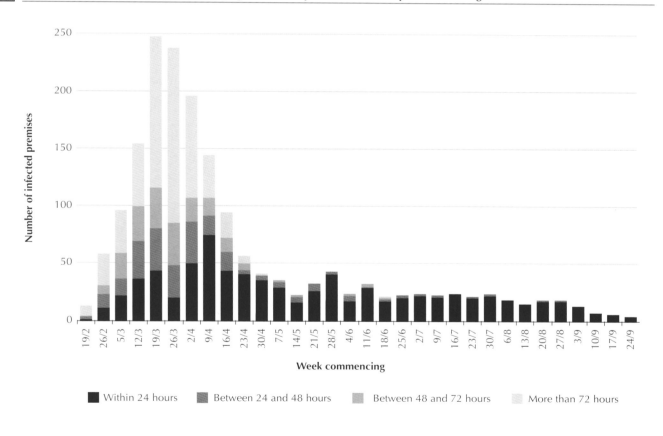

NOTE

The elapsed times shown are those between the slaughter of the last susceptible animal and disposal of the last animal.

Source: National Audit Office analysis of the records of 1,836 infected premises for which clear information was available on time between slaughter and disposal. The data was extracted from the Department's Disease Control System.

44 Animals slaughtered, disposed of and awaiting disposal by week during the 2001 outbreak

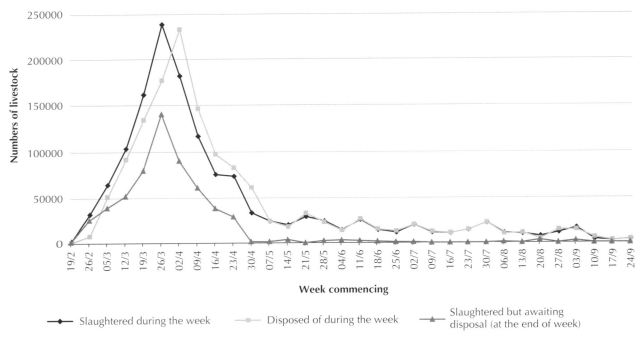

NOTE

The figures are for infected premises.

Source: National Audit Office analysis of data extracted from the Department's Disease Control System.

46 Main disposal methods used during the outbreak

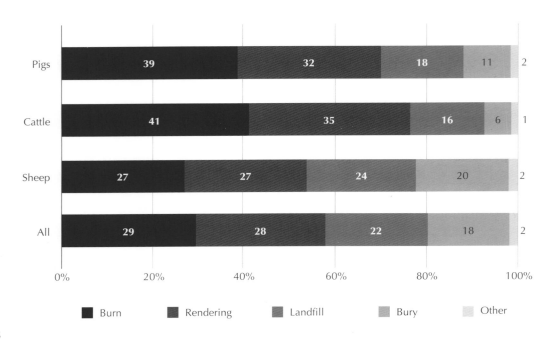

NOTES

1. The figures excludes animals slaughtered under the Livestock Welfare (Disposal) Scheme and in the three kilometre cull.
2. Burn includes incineration, on-farm burning and mass pyres.
3. Landfill includes mass burials.
4. Because of rounding numbers may not add up to 100.

Source: National Audit Office analysis of the Department's data.

totals for slaughtering had run ahead of disposals. On between a quarter and a third of infected premises, slaughtered animals were left lying on the ground for four days or more during these first seven weeks of the epidemic. As a result, the number of slaughtered animals awaiting disposal on infected premises increased rapidly, peaking at 140,000 on 1 April 2001 **(Figure 44)**. The number on dangerous contact premises peaked at 169,000 on 14 April 2001. The backlog was most serious in Devon, where it exceeded 100,000 carcasses.

3.97 The disposal rate lagged behind the slaughter rate until mid-April 2001, partly because of resource and logistical constraints. These included shortages of animal health officers and leak-proof transport for off-farm disposal along narrow country lanes. The scale of the operation also presented unprecedented challenges - on the peak day of 5 April 2001, more than 100,000 animals were disposed of for disease control purposes. By contrast, in 1967-68 the peak weekly disposal was 13,500 animals. Another main cause of the delay was a shortage of environmentally suitable and safe disposal sites.

3.98 The Department initially disposed of carcases through on-farm burial and burning, as it had done in 1967-68. This had the advantage of speed and minimisation of the risk of disease transmission. However, in many places these methods of disposal were not possible because of environmental constraints imposed by the Water Resources Act (1991), the Conservation Act (1994), and the Groundwater Regulations (1998). On-farm burial was also not practicable in areas with a thin layer of topsoil or where groundwater levels were unusually high following the wet autumn and winter, with consequent risks to controlled waters. In mid-March 2001, it was agreed that before each disposal the Environment Agency would conduct a rapid (within three-hours) groundwater site assessment and advise on an appropriate disposal method. A new preferred disposal hierarchy was also agreed with the Environment Agency on 15 March 2001 **(Figure 45)**. On

24 April 2001 the Department of Health issued guidance on how the risks to public health could be minimised, including the hierarchy of disposal options and advice on the location of pyres. The hierarchy took account of risks to the environment and human health. It was substantially different to the Department's initial approach as this had been focussed on animal health risks and logistical factors.

3.99 The disposal methods adopted took account of the preferred hierarchy and the circumstances of individual cases, for example, the availability of nearby rendering capacity, the relative risks of transferring carcasses over significant distances and the suitability of sites for burial or burning. The most commonly used methods during the whole epidemic were burning (29 per cent of carcasses), rendering (28 per cent), landfill (22 per cent) and burial (18 per cent) **(Figure 46)**.

45 | **Approved disposal routes for different species and age of stock**

Preferred Method of disposal	Permitted animals
1. Rendering	All
2. High-temperature incineration	All
3. Landfill, on approved sites	Sheep, pigs of any age and cattle born after 1 August 1996
4. Burning	All (with a limit of 1,000 cattle per pyre)
5. Mass burial or on-farm burial on approved sites	Sheeps, pigs of any age and cattle born after 1 August 1996

NOTE

1. Rendering or incineration were required options for cattle over five years' old

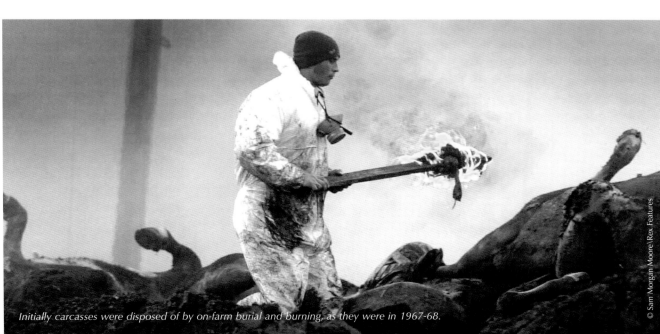

Initially carcasses were disposed of by on-farm burial and burning, as they were in 1967-68.

Nearly half a million carcasses were buried in a pit at Great Orton in Cumbria.

3.100 In practice the Department experienced problems with all the disposal methods used **(Figure 47)**. Rendering was not used until biosecurity protocols for rendering lorries and plants had been agreed. High-temperature incineration was rarely possible because the facilities capable of taking whole cattle carcasses were fully committed to the disposal of BSE-affected cattle. However, specially imported air-curtain incinerators were used on occasion. The use of landfill sites encountered resistance from some operators and from local communities, as many sites were near large urban centres. Because of these difficulties, many carcasses were disposed of in March 2001 on mass pyres. But this generated negative images in the media and had profound effects for the tourist industry. The Department considers that the problems with the various disposal options had not significantly contributed to delays in slaughter.

3.101 The backlog of slaughtered animals awaiting disposal built up to a peak of over 200,000 carcasses in early April 2001. Carcasses were sometimes left rotting on farms for days on end and this discouraged prompt slaughter, particularly for contiguous premises. After considering a number of options, the Department decided to carry out mass burials on sites with impermeable clay soils that were remote from residential properties but accessible to large vehicles. The armed services and the Department rapidly identified several hundred possible locations. The Environment Agency quickly assessed them and seven suitable sites **(Figure 48 opposite)** were agreed upon and brought into use, with the necessary infrastructure, such as special access roads, being built where needed. Some 1.3 million carcasses were disposed of in these mass burial sites - principally sheep from the contiguous and three kilometre culls. Technical problems, for example, carcass liquid seepage, and public protests prevented the greater use of some sites.

47 Disposal by rendering, landfill and mass pyres

Rendering: Although the environmentally preferred disposal option, rendering posed disease control risks if lorries used to carry carcasses to plants were inadequately sealed. It was used to dispose of 28 per cent of carcasses by number and 22 per cent (131,000 tonnes) by weight. Rendering plants were not widely available until 9 March 2001. Protocols for the biosecurity of vehicles and rendering plants were issued on 4 March 2001. On 19 March 2001 a further protocol set out which vehicles had been approved as acceptable for transporting carcasses to rendering plants. By 29 March 2001, six plants, with an overall weekly rendering capacity of 15,000 tonnes, were in operation: Torrington, Motherwell, Exeter, Lancaster, Bradford and Widnes. By late April 2001, it was the main disposal channel used. The UK Renderers' Association told us that rendering plants operated at barely 40 per cent of national capacity. However, at the peak time of requirement, sufficient rendering capacity was not available for all circumstances, hence the need for alternative disposal methods. By the later stages of the epidemic rendering capacity was available but the number of carcasses needing to be disposed of had reduced.

Landfill: Commercial landfill sites were used to dispose of a fifth of carcasses. They were a disposal option favoured by the Environment Agency, after rendering and incineration, since the sites had already been environmentally assessed. On 25 March 2001, the Agency reached agreement with the Environmental Services Association and the Department on provision of licensed landfill capacity for this purpose and eventually 111 suitable facilities were identified. In practice, 29 landfills were used to dispose of 95,000 tonnes of carcasses, including 69,000 tonnes in Cumbria. Local opposition to lorries carrying carcasses to the sites, operator opposition, cost and distance from sites of infection - with large landfill sites typically being near large urban centres - meant that landfill was less widely used than it might have been.

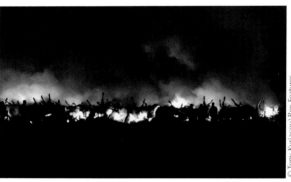

© Tony Kyriacou\Rex Features

Pyres: During March 2001, as disposal volumes increased, large pyres were used for carcass disposal. However, these led to negative media images and public opposition. On 7 May 2001 disposal via pyres was stopped. Over the course of the outbreak, around 30 per cent of carcasses were disposed of in burns, including 41 per cent of cattle. Burning took place on 950 sites, but most involved local on-farm burns. The largest concentrations of pyres were in southwest England, the Upper Severn, Cumbria and Wales.

48 **Mass burial sites identified and approved for carcass disposal**

Name	Location	Previous use	Area (hectares)	Date in 2001 when identified/ operational/ closed or received final carcasses	Potential capacity in terms of sheep carcasses (note 1)	Number of carcasses buried
Great Orton (Watchtree)	Cumbria	Airfield	209	23 March/ 26 March/ 7 May	750,000	460,000
Tow Law (Stonefoot Hill)	County Durham	Former open-cast coal working, used for heathland grazing	97	5 April/ 3 May/ 28 October	200,000	45,000
Widdrington (Seven Sisters)	Northumberland	Open-cast coal working that had been used for landfill	25	30 March/ 3 April/ 28 May	200,000	134,000
Throckmorton	Worcestershire	Open farmland	627	28 March/ 4 April/ 19 May	750,000	133,000
Birkshaw Forest	Dumfries and Galloway, Scotland	Commercial forest	50	26 March/ 29 March/ 25 May	1,000,000	490,000
Eppynt (Sennybridge)	Powys, Wales	Crown land adjacent to a clay quarry	17	28 March/ 5 April/ 14 April	300,000	0 (note 2)
Ash Moor	Devon	Fields and clay pits	41	15 March/ 2 May/ Mothballed on 14 May	350,000	0 (note 3)
Total					**3,550,000**	**1,262,000**

NOTES

1. On average a sheep weighed 50kg, a pig 100kg and cattle 500kg.

2. 18,000 carcasses were originally buried at Eppynt but because of seepage problems they were subsequently burnt, along with a further 19,500 carcasses.

3. By the time Ash Moor was opened, the need had passed.

Source: National Audit Office analysis of the Department's data.

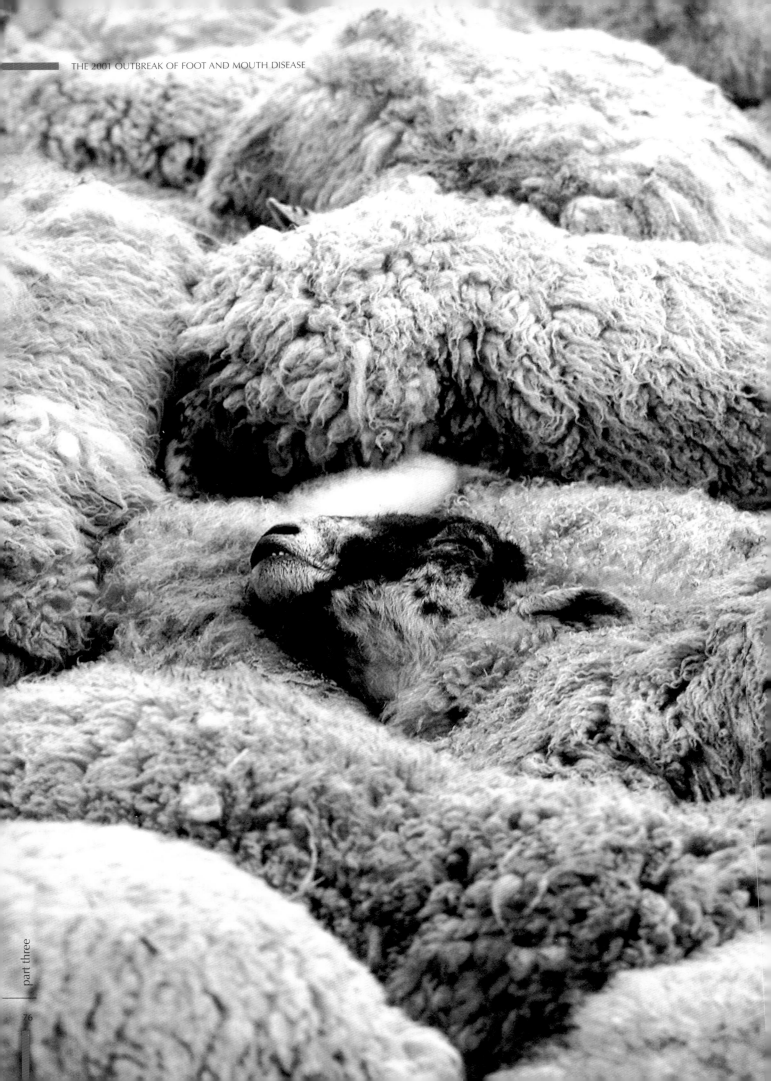

3.102 The significant efforts made by the Department, the military and others, such as the Environment Agency and the Scottish Environment Protection Agency, to build up disposal capacity and improve efficiency had a cumulative impact. By early May 2001, the backlog of carcasses awaiting disposal had been eliminated. There was now sufficient available capacity and by the end of the outbreak four of the seven mass burial sites were in fact used to less than a quarter of their capacities.

3.103 The disposal of carcasses was another hugely controversial issue throughout the 2001 outbreak and aroused the most public reaction. The use of mass burial and burn sites resulted in frequent demonstrations and community action to limit their use. Pyres of burning carcasses were vividly portrayed by the media and deterred overseas and domestic tourists from visiting the countryside. The Department's Interim Contingency Plan for dealing with foot and mouth disease in the future envisages the use of commercial incineration for the first few cases, with rendering then the preferred option and commercial landfill an alternative. The Department is negotiating a call-off agreement to provide for an assured minimum rendering capacity in any future outbreak. In the case of a major outbreak, structured agreements would be negotiated with national landfill sites. The Department has emphasised that it is unlikely that pyre burning or mass burial would be used again. However, the Department is awaiting the recommendations of the Lessons Learned and Royal Society Inquiries before any final decision is made.

Communications and information systems were severely stretched during the epidemic

'One of the lessons which is going to have to be looked at is how we communicate ... from the centre to local offices ... (from) local offices to farmers.. the sheer volume of communication that has to go on has to be seen to be believed ... and how do you get messages and information when things are changing so rapidly'. (Mr James Scudamore, Chief Veterinary Officer, speaking on 31 October 2001 before the House of Commons Select Committee on Environment, Food and Rural Affairs)

3.104 Effective communications are important to ensure that an accurate ground picture is obtained, that appropriate actions are taken and to build support and understanding among the parties involved. Although the Department had a range of electronic communications at its disposal that were not available in 1967-68, it proved difficult in crisis conditions for the Department to get its key instructions and messages across.

The volume of internal communications placed severe strains on Control Centre staff

3.105 The key elements of internal communications comprised:

- **Provision of guidance** from the headquarters to Disease Control Centres and to staff in the field. During the course of the outbreak, the Department's headquarters issued more than 500 Emergency Instructions, Action Notes and Field Information Notes to update staff on required operating procedures and to provide amendments to the veterinary field instruction manual. This information was disseminated via the Department's Intranet, but staff found it difficult to digest because of the pressure of work and because not all staff had access to computers. The difficulties in getting information across led to inconsistencies in approach between offices and meant that staff were not always up-to-date when handling queries from farmers and others. The Department regretted such a situation but considered it understandable given the circumstances. Rapid responses to the developing situation often required changes to instructions at very short notice. The Department is reviewing veterinary emergency instructions to ensure that they are presented in an easily digestible format and also include guidance for administrative and field staff.

- **Sharing information between offices** on good practice and cross-border activities. Information sharing between Disease Control Centres was patchy early on in the epidemic. As a consequence, expertise and lessons already learned were not shared as effectively as they could have been. There were also occasional breakdowns in communication. For example, there was a 10 day delay in the disposal of animals culled by the Worcester Disease Control Centre at Grosmont in Wales because the Cardiff Disease Control Centre had not been informed that the carcasses were ready to be collected for disposal. From April 2001 monthly meetings of Regional Operations Directors and Divisional Veterinary Managers were held to encourage sharing of information.

- **Provision of information on progress of the disease control campaign** from Disease Control Centres to headquarters (**Figure 49**). To make timely and appropriate decisions, Ministers, managers and scientific and veterinary advisers needed to be aware of emerging problems and have an accurate 'real time' picture of the situation on the ground in terms of resources available, actions taken and their impact. This was not always available because it took time for Disease Control Centres to gather up-to-date information from the field, input it and transmit it to headquarters. Headquarters was kept

49   The Disease Control System database

At the start of the outbreak, the Department had a State Veterinary Service Vetnet information technology database for recording livestock farm details. The 1999 Drummond Review of notifiable disease preparedness had identified gaps in coverage which meant that Vetnet 'could not be relied upon to provide an all embracing list of premises which would fall within infected area or surveillance zones'. Consequently, during the 2000 Classical Swine Fever Outbreak, a networked Disease Control System was built in prototype. This held information on infected and other premises, restrictions served, visits, and details of premises lying within Infected Areas. During the early weeks of the foot and mouth disease epidemic, the prototype was developed rapidly into a customised system, rolled-out to Disease Control Centres on 6 March 2001 and soon expanded to a system with several hundred concurrent users.

The Disease Control System became the core database during the epidemic, providing information on speed of slaughter and disposals that was fed into the daily statistical reports received by the Cabinet Office Briefing Room. It also provided some of the data used by the biomathematical modellers. Throughout March and April 2001 the reliability of some information was poor, particularly on the numbers of animals awaiting slaughter and disposal. Consequently, Disease Control Centres continued to use separate spreadsheets and databases that they had developed themselves. The system was gradually developed further and improved but problems persisted:

- **There were problems with data quality**: This arose from the work pressures on staff at Disease Control Centres and the lack of personnel on site available for data recording. Ongoing data cleansing led to removal of duplicated data in April 2001. However, checks in July 2001 showed there to be more than 800 affected premises with zero animals recorded against them. No dates were given for owner's reports of suspicions of disease for 95 of the more than 1,800 infected premises, while the date slaughtered was shown as before the owner's report date for 56 premises. The numbers of animals slaughtered also did not reconcile to that shown in the Department's compensation database. As late as December 2001, the Department issued an Emergency Instruction advising Disease Control Centres that over two thousand premises on the Disease Control System had map references ' located off the coast of Britain'.

- **Information was incomplete**: The Cabinet Office Briefing Room received incomplete daily speed to slaughter figures because Disease Control Centres lacked the resources to input this information rapidly. For example, in late May 2001, well past the peak of the epidemic, time to slaughter statistics provided by the Joint Co-ordination Centre for infected premises were based on less than two-thirds of the relevant cases. There were particular delays in inputting information to the Disease Control System on animals disposed of, sometimes because the relevant paper records were dispersed among the armed services and others. For example, the Disease Control System suggested on 7 April 2001 that 478,000 carcasses awaited disposal, whereas, in fact, the number was around 230,000.

informed of the disease situation via the field and headquarters epidemiology teams and daily situation reports from Disease Control Centres, setting out any extra resources required. Some difficulties in gaining an accurate picture of the situation on the ground contributed to personnel resources not being ramped up sufficiently quickly during the early weeks of the epidemic. There was an over-provision of disposal capacity from May 2001 because modelling predictions based on the information available in early April 2001 had suggested that twice as many carcasses were awaiting disposal than was actually the case. Based on this advice the Department considered it necessary to maintain an over-capacity for contingency reasons. The quality and timeliness of information provided to headquarters improved over time.

- **Keeping firms of contractors and other bodies assisting the Department appropriately** informed so as to co-ordinate their activities effectively. Respondents to our survey told us that arrangements were haphazard in some areas during the early weeks of the crisis. The Local Government Association said that initially communications and data sharing between the Department and local authorities were "very disappointing". The Environment Agency said that the Department's partners did not initially have a clear understanding of their respective roles and responsibilities in the crisis. Co-ordination of activities improved greatly from late March 2001, with the creation of the Joint Co-ordination Centre and the additional support received from the military.

The Department's external communications faced a severe challenge, though positive efforts were made to engage with external stakeholders

3.106 The Department spent £6 million on external communications during the outbreak. It also received assistance from other parts of government, including the Cabinet Office's News Co-ordination Centre, the devolved administrations (44 local information centres were set up in Wales) and the National Farmers' Union. It used a range of media, including the internet, call centres, distribution of leaflets and videos, advertising, meetings and media briefings **(Figure 50)**. The Department learned lessons, from the Phillips Inquiry into BSE, in being more open in communicating facts and analyses of risks. Lessons were also learned from the 1997 Mountfield Report on government communications during the late 1990s, with co-ordination and integration improved through daily conference calls between the foot and mouth disease Communications Director and regional press officers and the establishment of a Briefings Unit within the Joint Co-ordination Centre.

50 Timeline of the Department's external communication activities

Date in 2001	Cumulative number of infected premises	Development
20 February	1	The Department sets up a Foot and Mouth Disease Website and issues a press notice.
21 February	2	Daily press briefings begin.
22 February	3	The Department issues advice to farmers to operate to high hygiene standards and to the public to reduce contact with livestock and farms.
23 February	6	The Department sets up a national Foot and Mouth Disease Helpline and convenes the first of what were to become weekly, national stakeholder meetings. Twenty-nine trade organisations and interest groups are invited.
5 March	75	The Department sends out the first of what were to be 16 direct mailings to farmers, comprising advice on disease signs and on biosecurity.
March and April	31 to 1,518	The Foot and Mouth Disease Website attracts an average of 50,000 user sessions a day and calls to the helpline, which is available seven days a week and 24 hours a day, peak at 7,000 a day.
21 March	437	The Cabinet Office's News Co-ordination Centre provides information through its website. It was already providing a core brief three times a day. The Central Office of Information provides communications support to Disease Control Centres.
12 April	1,259	The Department sends out biosecurity advice leaflets to all livestock farmers.
6 July	1,814	The Department sends all livestock farmers a video and leaflet on biosecurity.

3.107 At a national level, the Department engaged stakeholders positively from 23 February 2001. This helped to alert it to emerging concerns and to improve stakeholder buy-in to agreed changes. A number of respondents to our survey, including the Food and Drink Federation, commended the Department's efforts in this respect.

3.108 Communications at a local level were less satisfactory initially. The Department provided a range of advice and support to affected farmers, through its website, helplines and direct mailings, while some Disease Control Centres set up local helplines and sent out newsletters. The National Farmers' Union felt that the website was a very valuable and generally well-designed channel of public communication. But it repeatedly had to exhort the Department to update the latest statistics on the website. The Department told us that providing foot and mouth statistics on its web site was treated as a priority and information on new cases was made available as soon as they were confirmed. The National Farmers' Union also said that not all farmers had internet access and during times of extreme pressure in local offices affected farmers sometimes found it difficult to contact staff as lines were engaged. It felt that many of the instances of misapplication of resources and delays in tackling problems and obstacles were rooted in failures in communications.

3.109 It is important that communications should be a two-way process. But on occasion the Department may not always have listened to or responded to local opinion. The Central Association of Agricultural Valuers told us that some local offices had shown little confidence in the potential contribution of local people and their knowledge. Local meetings of stakeholders were not always seen as a means for the local community to engage in a dialogue with the Department. The National Farmers' Union said that in some regions, especially in the early stages of the outbreak, there was no effective involvement of stakeholders who would have been able to contribute to the effort to combat the spread of the disease and to improve communications flows. The Department considers that in some regions, including the large Disease Control Centres in Carlisle and Leeds, local members of the National Farmers' Union played a very important liaison role bringing practical understanding of problems to the Disease Control Centre and helping to explain policy issues to farmers. The Devon Foot and Mouth Inquiry was persuaded that local knowledge was not sought and was dismissed when proffered. The Department has recognised that more needs to be done to involve local stakeholders and its Interim Contingency Plan envisages a more formalised structure for stakeholder involvement in the future.

3.110 Local communications improved once Regional Operations Directors were appointed. There were regular stakeholder meetings in most Disease Control Centres and good stakeholder involvement in the devolved administrations, building on strong local community structures. In Scotland this was particularly important in securing farmers' acceptance of the three kilometre and contiguous culls in Dumfries and Galloway, which checked the spread of the disease.

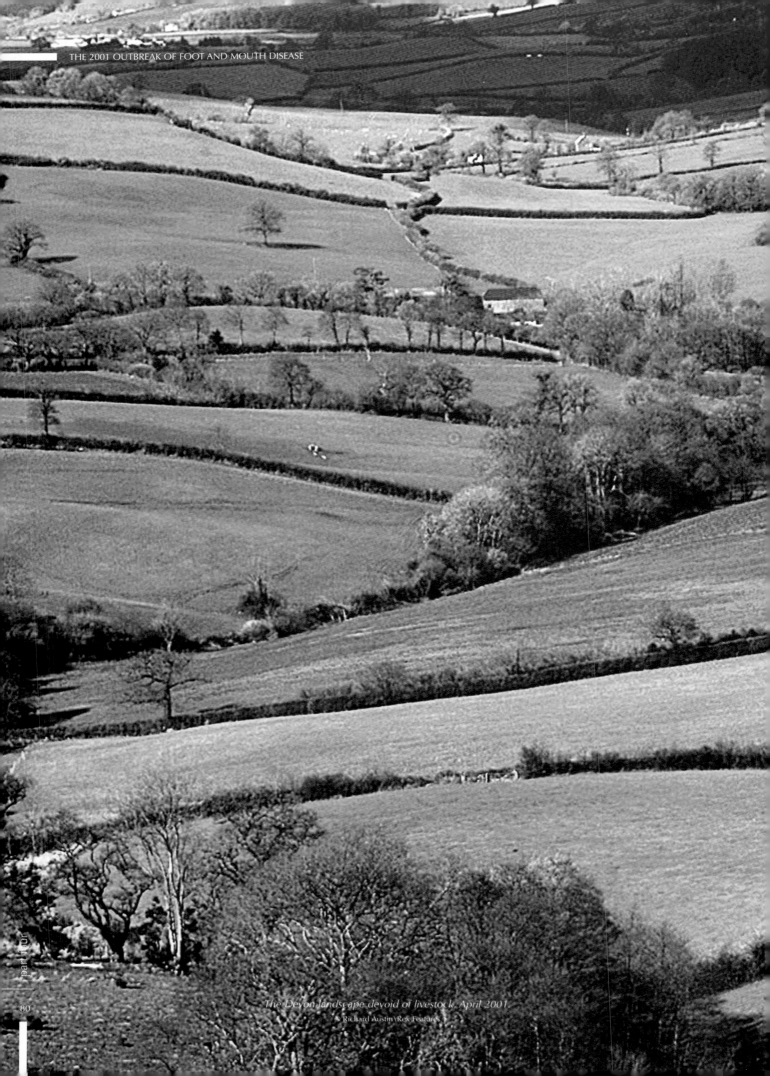

The Devon landscape devoid of livestock, April 2001.
© Richard Austin\Rex Features

Part 4

Controlling the costs of the outbreak

4.1 The Government's priority was to eradicate the disease with whatever resources were needed. Best value for money would be obtained by stamping the disease out quickly. The Department recognised that in the crisis conditions it was important to keep control of costs and to ensure that value for money was obtained.

4.2 This Part of the Report considers how well the Department controlled the costs of eradicating foot and mouth disease, taking into account the conditions under which it was operating at the time. We found that:

■ the Department and other government bodies are expected to spend over £3 billion dealing with the foot and mouth disease epidemic of 2001 (paragraph 4.4 and Figure 51);

■ there were difficulties in administering the compensation and payment schemes to farmers (paragraphs 4.5 to 4.34);

■ the procurement of services and supplies was costly and the Department was sometimes in a weak negotiating position (paragraphs 4.35 to 4.65); and

■ financial controls over payments were strengthened after initial problems (paragraphs 4.66 to 4.93).

4.3 Eradicating foot and mouth disease presented the Department with a tremendous logistical and supply chain challenge. A great many staff had to be brought together and a huge range of goods, services and works procured at short notice. This Herculean effort succeeded in bringing the disease under control, which was the main priority of the Government. At times, however, the Department and its staff were almost overwhelmed by the enormous flow of work. It was not surprising in these circumstances that existing systems of cost and financial control would be stretched almost to breaking point and that some mistakes would be made. It is therefore important in such circumstances that at least the bare minimum of basic controls should be in place. Such controls are needed both to prevent costs spiralling out of control, when it is not possible to follow normal tendering procedures, and to ensure that the Department pays only for the goods and services it has received. After the difficulties of the first few weeks the Department sought to strengthen cost and financial controls and to ensure that where mistakes were made they were corrected.

The Department and other government bodies are expected to spend over £3 billion dealing with the foot and mouth disease epidemic of 2001

4.4 Between the start of the outbreak in February 2001 and 24 May 2002 the Department and the Rural Payments Agency spent £1,341 million on compensation and payments to farmers. Over the same period the Department and other government bodies spent £1,074 million on measures to deal with the epidemic. The cost of the Department's and other Departments' staff time is estimated at £100 million. Support measures for businesses affected by the outbreak are estimated to have cost £282 million. And the Department calculates that it will need to spend a further £233 million on the outbreak and its aftermath. This will bring the total estimated bill for dealing with the epidemic to over £3 billion **(Figure 51)**.

There were difficulties in administering the compensation and payment schemes to farmers

The Department was legally required to compensate farmers for the slaughter of their animals

4.5 All farmers whose animals were slaughtered for disease control purposes were entitled to compensation as set out in Schedule 3 of the Animal Health Act, 1981. The Department also compensated farmers, in accordance with the requirements of the Act, for infected materials, such as straw, that were destroyed during the cull. The cost was huge - some £1,158 million - because

51 **Expenditure on foot and mouth disease by the Department, the Rural Payments Agency and other parts of Government**

Activity	Actual expenditure to 24 May 2002 (£ million)	Estimated likely final expenditure (£ million)
Payments to Farmers		
Compensation paid to farmers for animals culled and items seized or destroyed	1,130	1,158
Payments to farmers for animals slaughtered for welfare reasons[2]	211	211
Total payments to farmers	**1,341**	**1,369**
Direct costs of measures to deal with the epidemic		
Haulage, disposal and additional building work	252	375
Cleansing and disinfecting	295	304
Extra human resource costs	217	236
Administration of the Livestock Welfare (Disposal) Scheme, including operating costs, disposal charges and slaughter fees	164	164
Payments to other Government departments, local authorities, agencies and others	73	89
Miscellaneous, including serology, slaughtermen, valuers, equipment and vaccine	68	81
Claims against the Department	5	30
Total direct costs of measures to deal with the epidemic	**1,074**	**1,279**
Other costs		
Cost of the Department's and other government departments' staff time	100	100
Support measures for businesses affected by the outbreak[3]	282	282
Total other costs	**382**	**382**
TOTAL ALL COSTS	**2,797**	**3,030**

NOTES

1. All costs are provisional pending completion of a Departmental project to investigate the full cost of the outbreak.

2. Includes payments of £205.4 million under the Livestock Welfare (Disposal) Scheme and £5.3 million under the Light Lambs Scheme.

3. Includes £156 million available under European Union market support measures for agri-monetary compensation in respect of currency movements.

Source: Department for Environment, Food and Rural Affairs

compensation had to be paid in respect of 4.2 million animals that were slaughtered. Individual farmers received payments ranging from £20 to over £4 million (**Figure 52**). The average payment was around £125,000. The Department emphasises that, while individual payments appear high, livestock represented most farmers' livelihood.

Problems with the slaughter compensation scheme increased the Department's costs

Values of slaughtered animals

4.6 The average value for each type of livestock animal increased during the crisis, peaked and gradually declined. Figure 53 below shows the average value for cattle and sheep on a week by week basis. The average values for cattle rose from about £500 in the first four weeks of the crisis to about £1,500 at their peak in May 2001. Values then fell back to an average of £1,200 in September 2001. Average sheep values rose steadily from £100 in the first four weeks to £300 in July 2001 and then gradually declined.

4.7 The Animal Health Act 1981 requires compensation to be based on the value of the animal immediately before it became infected by foot and mouth disease. For animals exposed to infection, but not formally diagnosed as infected, compensation is based on the value of the animal immediately before slaughter. The word "value" in the Animal Health Act 1981 is not defined, although the Department's interpretation is that compensation would be based on "market" value and not, for example, on loss of future income. "Market values" were referred to on the departmental forms that valuers were required to use.

52 **Compensation payments received by farmers for the slaughter of livestock and destruction of infected materials in connection with the eradication of foot and mouth disease**

Size of compensation payment received

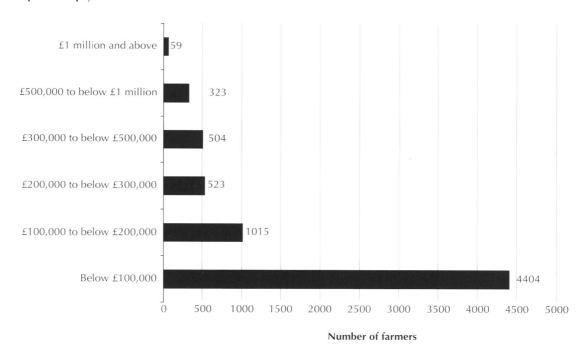

Number of farmers

NOTE

Farmers submitted more than 13,000 individual claims for destroyed animals and infected materials. This figure aggregates these claims by individual farmers. In total, claims were submitted by more than 6,800 individual farmers, as some farmers owned several separate premises where animals were slaughtered for disease control purposes.

Source: The Department's database for compensation payments, for payments up to 10 April 2002.

4.8 During the crisis professional valuers determined the value of the animal for the payment of compensation. They faced substantial practical difficulties in doing so because, as there were no freely functioning markets, valuers did not have any current prices to guide them, especially for breeding stock. As in 1967-68, valuations tended to rise during the course of the outbreak because valuers expected the resulting shortage of stock to be reflected in increased prices when the markets opened again. The Department told us that there were also inconsistencies in the way similar animals were valued, some prices being probably based on higher re-stock values. The Central Association of Agricultural Valuers[25] told the Department in June 2001 that in a minority of cases values for livestock were set "well above what was proper". The Department has investigated a number of such cases (see paragraph 4.15 below).

4.9 Valuation for animal disease control purposes is not straightforward and other Member States of the European Union have also encountered difficulties. For example, the European Commission reduced a claim by the Netherlands in respect of the costs of eradicating classical swine fever in 1998. The Netherlands are challenging in the European Court of Justice the Commission's assertion that too high a value was placed on swine.

Appointment of valuers

4.10 Livestock valuation is a specialised task requiring experts to undertake it. Only a small number of valuers in Britain have expertise in pedigree animals, individual herds, or other specialist stock. To aid the selection of valuers the Central Association of Agricultural Valuers provided a list of some 200 livestock valuers for the State Veterinary Service to use. Each Animal Health Divisional Office also maintained a list of valuers in its area. In Scotland lists of valuers were provided by the Institute of Auctioneers and Appraisers in Scotland.

4.11 Valuers were engaged by the Department. In practice, however, farmers were allowed to select a valuer of their choice from the local lists. The Department allowed farmers to choose their own valuer both to encourage co-operation with early slaughter to eradicate the disease and to reduce the chances of any disputes. But as a result:

■ Some valuers may not have had the expertise or qualifications to value all classes of animals. The Central Association of Agricultural Valuers told us that some farmers chose, for example, officials of breed societies, cattle dealers and others who may not have been suitable, especially for pedigree animals.

part four

25 *The main professional body representing valuers in England and Wales.*

53 **Average valuations for slaughtered cattle and sheep over the course of the outbreak**

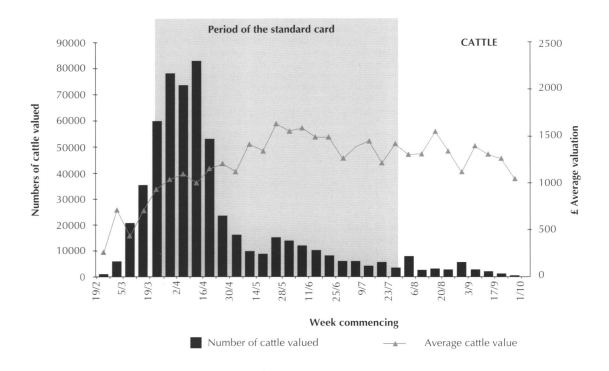

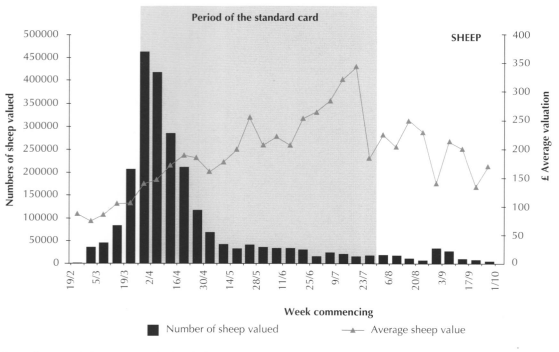

Source: Department for Environment, Food and Rural Affairs

■ It was usual for the valuer to be local and known to the farmer. Local farmers would have been aware of the valuations being made and some may have shopped around to secure the most favourable valuations. The Central Association of Agricultural Valuers considered this a very "corrosive practice" that put professional valuers under great pressure.

4.12 The Northumberland Report on the 1967-68 outbreak of foot and mouth disease found that prices had risen during the crisis and identified similar difficulties in valuing animals. The Report recommended that senior valuers should be appointed by the Department on a regional basis to monitor valuations and to help to secure uniformity. The Department's standing instructions for veterinary staff envisaged the appointment of senior valuers, but in the event no steps were taken by the Department to appoint such valuers until July 2001, when advisers were appointed to look at valuations and provide weekly reports on prices.

Payment of fees to valuers

4.13 The Department expects to pay £10 million in fees to valuers. The fee structure was agreed after discussions between the Department and the Central Association of Agricultural Valuers. It was designed to be simple so as to minimise delays in valuation and slaughter to prevent the spread of the disease. Fees were based on one per cent of the value of the stock dealt with, with a minimum fee of £500 a day and a maximum fee of £1,500 a day irrespective of the number of animals that were valued. The Department considers that capping the daily fee regardless of the number of animals involved or their value helped to address the possibility that a valuer might have an interest in overvaluing animals. The average compensation payment was £125,000 and the £1,500 a day cap applied in around 17 per cent of cases. Nevertheless, a scheme that links fees to the size of valuation is inherently risky and open to abuse. The Department is investigating one allegation of malpractice (paragraph 4.77) but considers that there has not been widespread abuse.

4.14 In May 2001 the Central Association of Agricultural Valuers advised the Department that in its opinion the £1,500 a day cap was set too low partly because at the start of the outbreak when the fees were negotiated it was not envisaged that there might be several valuations on infected premises that might run before dawn into the night. The Association also argued that a valuer was prevented from valuing for five days after visiting an infected premises and might therefore have to forego other income he or she could have earned from valuations elsewhere. The valuation exercise was also undertaken outside normal working hours and under distressing conditions. The Department considered the request but decided not to increase the rates.

Checks on exceptionally high compensation payments

4.15 Very high valuations were made on some of the pedigree animals that were culled. **Figure 54** shows the highest compensation amounts paid for individual animals. Where it appeared that a valuation was fundamentally flawed, the Department took steps to establish whether that valuation was in fact reasonably representative of market value. Many of the animals slaughtered during the epidemic were indisputably of high value. The Department therefore had the task of ascertaining what the appropriate level of payment for pedigree animals should be. The Department's finance branch is continuing to review high valuations and seek justification for them from valuers. In some cases the Department did not find the evidence - such as bloodlines and prices paid for the animals - to support the claims made for pedigree animals. By April 2002, the Department had written to more than 150 valuers asking for evidence to support their valuations. Some of these cases remain under investigation and some payments have been held up but, to date, no valuations have been reduced.

54 **Highest compensation payments for slaughtered animals as at mid May 2002**

Animal	Highest value
Cattle	£48,000 for a pedigree Limousin bull
Sheep	£50,000 for a Swaledale ram
Pig	£20,000 for a pure-bred seven year old wild boar
Deer	£50,000 for a stag

Source: The Department for Environment, Food and Rural Affairs.

The attempt to set standard rates for compensation contributed to a rise in prices

4.16 On 20 March 2001, Ministers agreed that urgent action was needed to secure speedier valuations of animals subject to compulsory slaughter. The valuation process was thought to be delaying the slaughter of animals on infected premises and it was hoped that introducing a standard valuation card would speed things up. To remove the need for a formal valuation, livestock keepers would be offered payment at standard rates for slaughtered animals, though farmers would have the right to refuse the standard valuation and have their animals valued by a valuer.

4.17 The standard rate card was introduced on 22 March 2001. To encourage its use the standard rates were intended to be generous, being pitched within the highest quartile of market prices before the February 2001 outbreak (as provided by the Meat and Livestock Commission). The rates ranged from £150 to £1,100 for cattle, from £32 to £150 for sheep, and from £18 to £520 for pigs. The Department expected that at least 70 per cent of farmers whose animals were to be slaughtered would accept the standard payment rates rather than seek individual valuations.

4.18 In fact the standard rates were used by only 4 per cent of farmers. Most chose to appoint a valuer. But the standard rate card contributed to a rise in valuations. The average valuation of cattle rose from £905 when the card was introduced to £1,300 in July 2001; the valuation of sheep rose from £100 to £210 over the same period. Some increase was expected as the standard rates were introduced to encourage rapid agreement to slaughter. Stocks of animals were also declining. However, the standard rates acted as a floor for valuations and contributed to "valuation creep". Farmers might choose to have standard valuations for their poor and average quality animals but obtain separate and higher valuations for their better quality stock.

4.19 In June and early July 2001, the Department reviewed the standard rate valuation system. The Department concluded that, with the changing seasons, the rates no longer covered relevant categories of animals such as new season lambs. The Department also concluded that the rates may have been acting to increase valuations and that the conditions which led to their introduction at the height of the epidemic no longer prevailed. The standard rates were therefore abolished with effect from 30 July 2001.

4.20 By April 2002, the Department had received a total of 1,430 complaints and disputes about valuations. The disputes were generally from farmers who complained that their valuations were low when compared to those obtained by their neighbours for similar types of animal. Another main area of dispute was that farmers claimed that the standard rates, introduced on 22 March 2001, should have been backdated to the start of the outbreak. These standard rates were often higher than the values farmers had previously received from valuers before this date.

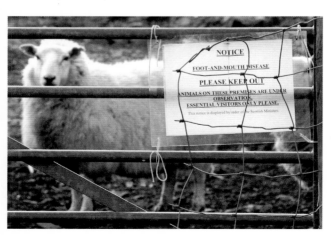

4.21 The Department is currently reviewing two aspects of the valuation procedures in the light of the lessons learned from the foot and mouth disease outbreak of 2001. The first review is examining the appointment and monitoring of valuers. The second review is investigating a sample of compensation cases to analyse the factors affecting stock valuations during the 2001 outbreak.

The Livestock Welfare (Disposal) Scheme helped many farmers but the generous rates created demand that exceeded initial capacity

4.22 On 22 March 2001 the Department introduced the Livestock Welfare (Disposal) Scheme. This voluntary scheme was intended to alleviate the suffering of animals who were not directly affected by foot and mouth disease but could not be moved to alternative accommodation or pasture nor sent to market because of movement restrictions. For example, as pigs are normally moved to slaughter or new accommodation on a weekly basis and new piglets are born each week, overcrowding of accommodation could quickly occur.

4.23 Under the Livestock Welfare (Disposal) Scheme, farmers received payment for the slaughter of eligible animals. The Rural Payments Agency ran the scheme on behalf of the Department, the Scottish Executive and the National Assembly for Wales. The State Veterinary Service and local veterinary inspectors provided any necessary welfare inspections and certifications, while a team of consultants from ADAS Consulting Ltd assisted from the outset with the prioritisation of applications and fast tracking of those cases that appeared most urgent. Under the scheme, the Rural Payments Agency paid farmers £205 million for the slaughter of two million animals at more than 18,000 farms and collection points. The scheme cost £164 million to run, including operating costs, disposal charges, slaughter fees and administration.

The rates for animals were generous

4.24 Payments made to farmers under the scheme were not compensation payments and therefore did not have to reflect the value of the animals killed. The payment rates for the scheme were initially set at levels which were up to 90 per cent of the standard rate values, ranging from £22 for a non-breeding ewe to £900 for a breeding cow. The Rural Payments Agency also met the cost of transporting the animals to slaughter. The rates were agreed between Ministers and farmers' leaders on the understanding that the rates would be reviewed within two months.

4.25 In setting up the scheme the Department expected that farmers would pursue all other means of retaining or marketing their animals and turn to the scheme only as a last resort. This did not always happen, however. The rates were extremely attractive to farmers and generally considered to be higher than the market price would have been if markets had been operating. At a discussion of the Cabinet Office Briefing Room in early April 2001, it was noted that the level of payments was providing incentives to farmers to let their livestock become welfare problems. Due to the large number of claims with modest or no welfare problems, claims from some farmers with serious immediate problems took longer to process than the State Veterinary Service would have wished. In short, the high rates were subverting the objectives of the scheme, which was failing in its original purpose of alleviating animal suffering.

4.26 Some rates were reduced in April 2001 and more substantial reductions were made in July 2001 and October 2001. For example, in July 2001 the rate for breeding cows was reduced to £700 for those aged up to four years and to £350 for those over four years old. The rate for sows was reduced from £75 per head to £30 per head. The rate reductions are being challenged in the courts by the National Farmers' Union because the Department reduced the payments after six weeks rather than the two months proposed in March 2001.

Demand for the scheme was initially heavy and backlogs built up

4.27 Between March and December 2001 the Rural Payments Agency received over 18,000 applications to slaughter some 3,100,000 animals. In the first two weeks of the scheme nearly 5,000 applications were received and over one million animals were registered under the scheme. A large backlog of applications built up. By mid May 2001, some 335,000 animals registered with the scheme had not been slaughtered. There were several problems:

- The initial volume of applications overwhelmed the Agency. There were insufficient staff to deal with applications and requests for information from farmers. The situation was exacerbated because a large volume of applications in the first few weeks - representing 876,000 animals - were duplicates.

- There was a lack of facilities for the disposal of slaughtered animals because diseased animals were given priority. It was a principle of the scheme that no animal would be collected unless a confirmed slaughter and disposal route was available. When the scheme was introduced in March 2001 only one rendering plant was available for the scheme; and it took 10 days before commercial landfill sites were available, mainly because site operators were not equipped to begin operation as early as they had initially indicated. Some sites which entered into agreements to take material later withdrew due to local opposition. In addition some were seeking exceptionally high rates. The problem was particularly acute in Wales in the first few weeks because, while eight landfill sites were approved by the Environment Agency from the outset, the owners of the sites were reluctant to enter into contracts with the Rural Payments Agency because of local opposition.

4.28 Some animals with genuine welfare problems died before they could be collected for slaughter. Others had to wait up to six weeks before removal. The Royal Society for the Prevention of Cruelty to Animals told us that the suffering of some animals on farms was such that in normal circumstances the Society would have prosecuted under the Protection of Animals Act 1911. In cases where animals died before slaughter, the farmer was not entitled to any payment.

4.29 Over one million animals were slaughtered during the first seven weeks of the scheme. The backlog of animals was gradually reduced: more administrators were employed; the logistics of veterinary tasks, disposal and transportation were better co-ordinated; and more facilities for disposal, such as landfill sites, became available. Ninety telephone lines were installed at the Rural Payments Agency's offices to help with inquiries from farmers. Demand for the Scheme reduced as movement restrictions were eased and financial incentives were reduced.

There were problems over eligibility

4.30 Only animals with immediate welfare problems or those likely to develop in the ensuing four weeks were eligible under the Scheme. In preparing the eligibility criteria the Department was aware that there would be limited government veterinary or animal health resources available to scrutinise applications, inspect premises, check records and verify claims. Proper operation of the scheme therefore depended in part on the honesty of applicants. However, from the start of the scheme all applications had to be supported by a statement from the farmer's private veterinary surgeon. Applications were prioritised for slaughter by a team of advisers from ADAS Consulting Ltd contracted to the Department. From early May 2001 the role of ADAS Consulting Ltd was expanded to include specific eligibility checks on individual farms, local movement restrictions and stocking densities. Evidence of the farmer's efforts to obtain movement licences, secure additional grazing and/or sell stock was required before an application could be accepted. Prior to slaughter a local veterinary inspector employed by the Department was required to carry out an inspection to corroborate the facts presented by the farmer and his or her private vet.

4.31 There were a number of administrative problems with the scheme:

- Although 14,000 applications were accepted, over 3,000 applications in respect of over one million animals were either rejected by the Agency or later withdrawn by farmers because they did not meet the eligibility criteria. The administrative effort required to scrutinise these applications deflected attention from processing eligible claims.

- Because veterinary resources were limited, private vets may sometimes have endorsed an application without seeing the animals or simply on the basis of a telephone conversation with the farmer, particularly where the animals were in the care of a private veterinary surgeon who was familiar with the enterprise and the current problems. It is therefore possible that, if farmers provided incorrect information to their private vets, some applications with ineligible animals may have been supported. The inspection by a local veterinary inspector prior to slaughter sought to deal with the possibility that ineligible animals might be claimed for.

- Some of the eligibility criteria were not sufficiently well defined when the Scheme was set up. It was unclear, for example, whether a "breeding cow" merely needed to be capable of breeding or had to have given birth. There was also uncertainty over cases where farmers claimed to be in ill health and could not tend their animals. This lack of clarity caused confusion among farmers and vets and may have led to incorrect claims being made. Such incorrect claims could not have been picked up without inspecting the animals concerned.

4.32 Once the backlog of cases had begun to reduce, the Department was able to consider interim changes to the administration of the scheme. Changes were made on 30 April 2001: eligibility criteria were clarified, applications underwent greater scrutiny and some payment rates were reduced. There then followed a consultation exercise on the need for further changes to the scheme. Following the consultation exercise, the Livestock Welfare (Disposal) Scheme was closed to new applicants on 27 July 2001 and replaced by a new scheme with effect from 30 July 2001. The main changes included:

- reduced payment rates to reflect the increasing options available to farmers as disease restrictions were eased;

- limiting the number of animals that could be entered into the scheme to a maximum of 30 per cent of the total livestock on a farm holding; and

- better guidance to farmers and vets as to how eligibility under the scheme would be assessed.

From 1 January 2002 applicants received no money, just the disposal of their animals at no charge. The scheme ceased completely at the end of February 2002.

Many farmers and rural businesses suffered consequential losses

4.33 Farmers whose animals did not have foot and mouth disease, were not deemed at risk, or were not suffering from poor welfare conditions were not entitled to any payment. European Union regulations prohibited such aid. For example, around 130,000 farms, where livestock could not be moved because they were subject to Infected Area restrictions, fell into this category. Yet they could suffer greater financial hardship than farmers who met the criteria for payments because they had no extra income to meet the additional costs of providing food for animals that had to be retained on their farms for long periods. The Department has estimated that the outbreak cost agricultural producers £355 million after taking account of compensation and other payments to farmers. Some £175 million of this cost was incurred as a result of the restrictions on animal movements.

4.34 Many rural businesses were also badly affected by the outbreak as they were not entitled under the Animal Health Act 1981 to compensation for consequential losses. The Government introduced a series of measures to alleviate the financial difficulties of small businesses. These included the deferral of tax and VAT payments (around £242 million in tax was deferred for periods of up to two years); increases in rate relief for businesses facing hardship (over £20 million); extension of the Small Firm Loan Guarantee Scheme (an extra £120 million in additional loans were made available); extra funds for the Business Recovery Fund (over £50 million); and a charity matching scheme whereby the government matched donations given by the public to voluntary organisations to relieve hardship caused by the outbreak. In addition £156 million was available under European Union market support measures for agri-monetary compensation in respect of currency movements. The Scottish Executive and the National Assembly for Wales have also provided funding packages to help businesses to recover from the effects of foot and mouth disease.

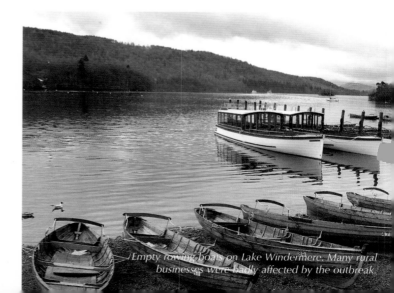

Empty rowing boats on Lake Windermere. Many rural businesses were badly affected by the outbreak.

The procurement of services and supplies was costly and the Department was sometimes in a weak negotiating position

Goods and services were purchased from a range of private and public sector organisations

4.35 The Department and the Rural Payments Agency had spent by 24 May 2002 over £1,100 million on goods and services to eradicate the disease (Figure 51 on page 82). The total bill for measures to deal with the epidemic is expected to reach nearly £1,300 million by the time all claims have been settled. Payments have been made to over 1,200 firms of contractors, ranging from small local firms to national and multinational combines. Major firms involved included some of the largest transport and construction companies in Britain **(Figure 55)**. Middle ranking and smaller local firms also made a substantial contribution. They supplied local transport and labour, the materials required to burn pyres, and local services such as animal slaughter, animal valuation, legal services and veterinary inspection.

4.36 Payments were also made to farmers and other groups. Farmers have received about 40 per cent of the £295 million paid out to date for cleansing and disinfecting their farms. Landfill site operators received substantial sums for receiving slaughtered animals. Landowners were paid several million pounds for allowing their land to be used as mass burial sites. The Department also contracted goods and services from other government departments, executive agencies, local authorities and the police.

Some of the goods and services required were inherently expensive

The need for speed

4.37 The Department's overriding priority was to eradicate the disease. Ministers issued instructions that any obstacles to achieving this objective must be removed. Speed was paramount and cost was of secondary importance. Ministers believed that best value for money would be achieved by eradicating the disease as quickly as possible.

55 **Firms of contractors in receipt of the highest payments**

Contractor	Main areas of operation	Payments received to 23 May 2002 (£ million)
Snowie Limited	Transport and equipment in Scotland; transport, equipment, disposal and burial pit construction in Northern England	38.4
JDM Midlands Limited	Cleansing and disinfecting in Worcester, Gloucester and Devon	27.5
ADAS Consulting Limited	Consultancy advice, cleansing and disinfecting supervision, vaccination preparation and management of the long-distance movement scheme	24.1
Carillion	Site disposal and operation and management of fixed facilities in the North East and Cumbria	21.1
Cumbria Waste Management Limited	Disposal, transportation and landfill sites in Cumbria	17.5
Greyhound Plant Services	Disposal and transportation in Wales	14.4
Barr Limited	Supervision, labour, plant and transportation in connection with burn sites, including ash disposal and burial pit construction in Scotland	14.3
Midas Construction	Disposal and transportation in Devon, the Midlands and Wales	11.4
Whitkirk Produce Company Limited	Transport and cleansing and disinfecting	9.9
Dumfries and Galloway Council	Cleansing and disinfecting, burns and burials, management of emergency operations centre in Dumfries	9.9

NOTE

Payment figures are exclusive of VAT.

Source: The Department for Environment, Food and Rural Affairs

4.38 The Department recognised that it would have to pay a premium to get things done at maximum possible speed. Thus, for example, the Department spent much more on the construction of burial pits for slaughtered animals than it would have done had the task not been so urgent. The firms that constructed these pits worked 24 hours a day, seven days a week to meet the Department's tight deadlines and this substantially increased the expenditure on overtime, night-time and weekend working. Burial site construction on the scale required would normally have taken two years.

Shortages of goods and services

4.39 The crisis conditions quickly led to shortages of equipment and materials and it was also difficult to find firms to undertake various services. The Department had little or no control over this. When the outbreak started many local firms were reluctant to assist in the crisis. Some thought that they would be tarnished by association with animal slaughter in connection with foot and mouth disease and that they would lose agricultural contracts in the future. In Devon, for example, local contractors were reluctant to get involved. Much of the work involved in containing the outbreak - slaughter, disposal and cleansing in particular - was difficult, dirty and potentially hazardous. In these circumstances it was inevitable that some contractors would demand higher prices than under normal conditions.

4.40 Because of the shortages, the Department may have paid significantly more for the materials required to eradicate the disease. Wooden railway sleepers needed for pyres were bought in February and March 2001 for between £5 and £20 each. By October 2001 the Department estimated that the value of some 100,000 unused sleepers had fallen to between £1 and £10 each; and the amount realisable would be significantly less as the Department would also have to pay the transportation costs. The price paid for coal was anything up to £130 a tonne. Surplus stocks are now worth less than £15 a tonne, partly because some of the coal had been contaminated with small rocks.

Environmental and health considerations

4.41 Substantial costs were incurred in protecting the environment and public health. Some of the highest costs were in respect of the disposal of slaughtered animals. In 1967-68 many of the laws that now protect the environment did not exist. In 1967-68 on-farm burial and pyre burning were used extensively, at almost negligible cost. In 2001 on-farm burial was generally not used because the water table in many parts of the country was too high and this increased the risks of controlled waters being affected.

4.42 Considerable costs were incurred on the construction of burial pits in March and April 2001. The Department acquired the land for seven mass burial pits: five in England, one in Scotland and one in Wales. These pits were an entirely new form of engineering and had to be designed from scratch. Most pits took less than a week to bring into operation. The Department had to invest heavily in measures to deal with environmental concerns, such as the possible release of leachate (animal body fluids) into watercourses, contaminated surface water and the disposal of contaminants. At Great Orton in Cumbria, for example, a wall three miles long was constructed at a cost of £3.5 million (including VAT) as a further safeguard to ensure that there was no contamination of ground water.

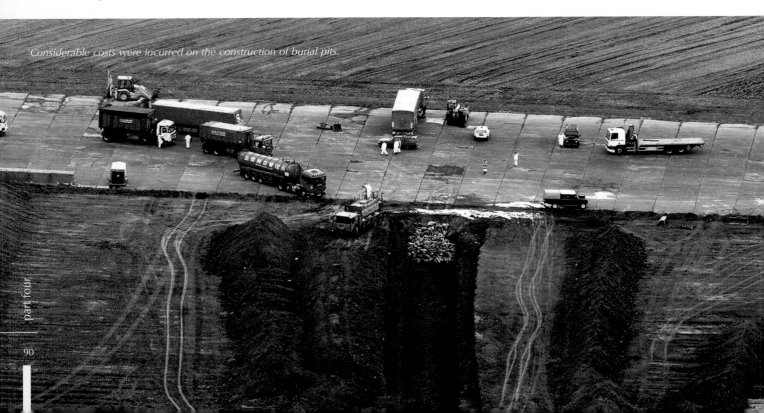

Considerable costs were incurred on the construction of burial pits.

4.43 The total cost of purchasing and building the mass burial pits up until 31 March 2002 was £79 million. Further costs will be incurred to restore, monitor and maintain these sites, in some cases for the next 15 years. Costs of restoration and management in the future are estimated at £35 million, which will bring the total cost of the sites to £114 million (**Figure 56**). Many sites have little resale value. No decisions have yet been taken on the future of the burial sites.

4.44 The mass burial sites were used to about only one-third of their capacity (Figure 48 on page 75) for two main reasons:

- **Technical problems:** Eppynt, in Wales, could not be used for permanent burial. The Environment Agency and local authorities had carried out rapid geological and environmental assessments of the site before a burial pit was constructed. However, in the short time available the assessments were not sufficiently probing and, six days after the site opened, leachate was found in a borehole 100 yards away. The site was temporarily suspended and later closed and 18,000 carcasses that had been buried in the pit had to be exhumed and burnt at a cost of some £2.2 million.

56 Expenditure on mass burial pits

1. Burial site	2. Purchase costs (£m)		3. Construction, operation and maintenance costs to 31 March 2002 (£m)	4. Estimated costs of restoration and site maintenance from 2002-03 to end of life (£m)	5. Likely total costs to the Department (£m)	6. Number of carcasses permanently buried
	Freehold land purchase	Rent for term of lease				
Great Orton (Watchtree), Cumbria	3.2	0.6	17.9	13.4	35.1	460,000
Tow Law (Stonefoot Hill), County Durham	0.5[1]	-	7.6	7.1	15.2	45,000
Widdrington (Seven Sisters), Northumberland	0.3	0.2	3.2	1.4	5.1	134,000
Throckmorton, Worcestershire	3.9	-	11.4	7.3	22.6	133,000
Birkshaw Forest, Dumfries and Galloway, Scotland	0.5	-	5.0	4.5	10.0	490,000
Eppynt, (Sennybridge) Powys, Wales	-	Held rent-free as located on Crown land.	18.5	0.4	18.9	0[2]
Ash Moor, Devon	0.3	-	5.5	1.2	7.0	0[3]
Total	**8.7**	**0.8**	**69.1**	**35.3**	**113.9**	**1,262,000**

NOTES

1. Includes £165,000 paid to UK Coal in compensation for coal that could not be mined because of the buried carcasses.

2. 18,000 carcasses were buried at Eppynt but because of seepage problems they were subsequently exhumed and burnt. An additional 19,500 carcasses were imported to the site and were also burnt. The data include costs for burial, exhumation, burning and ash removal.

3. By the time Ash Moor was opened, the need had passed.

Source: the Department, the Scottish Executive and the National Assembly for Wales.

■ **Overprovision of capacity:** The Department overestimated the number of carcasses that needed to be disposed of for mass burial. This was partly because, when decisions to build mass burial sites were taken, the outbreak's course and the availability of other disposal routes remained uncertain. With hindsight, the decline in daily confirmed cases turned out to be sharper than the Department had prepared for. Ash Moor in Devon, for example, was never used for mass burial, because a 'flare up' of the disease in Dartmoor, which the Department had feared, did not occur.

4.45 Dealing with the ash from pyres also proved expensive because of the care with which it had to be disposed of. In 1967-68 the ash from pyres was buried on farms at negligible cost. In 2001 there were concerns about the safe disposal of the ash and on-farm burial was generally considered not to be a satisfactory option **(Figure 57)**. Some 120,000 tonnes of ash had therefore to be disposed of in landfill sites, at a cost of £38 million.

57 **Disposing of the ash from pyres**

Almost all the pyres included cattle over five years old and there was a potential risk of Bovine Spongiform Encephalopathy (BSE) infectivity. Initially the assumption had been that the ash would be buried on site, and in some cases this happened. But where the groundwater table was high or particularly large number of carcasses had been burnt, the Environment Agency advised against on-site burial. In May 2001 a Working Group of the Spongiform Encephalopathy Advisory Committee, set up to consider the risks of ash disposal, noted that high temperature incineration or burial in landfill sites were suitable options for disposal. Incineration was relatively expensive at over £500 a tonne and the Committee estimated that it would take 8-10 years to dispose of an estimated 100,000 tonnes of ash. Where necessary the Environment Agency modified the conditions of landfill site licences to enable particular types of waste to be disposed of.

Because of the crisis situation the Department had to pay over the odds for some goods and services

4.46 Some of the problems faced by the Department in keeping costs under control are illustrated by the case study of cleansing and disinfecting at **Figure 58**.

The Department was sometimes in a weak negotiating position

4.47 The need for speed in eradicating the disease, and the general shortage of goods and services, put the Department in a relatively weak position to negotiate contracts and set fee rates for key services. Without valuers, slaughterers and private vets, for example, the disease could not have been eradicated. All demanded and received higher fee rates. For example, slaughterers

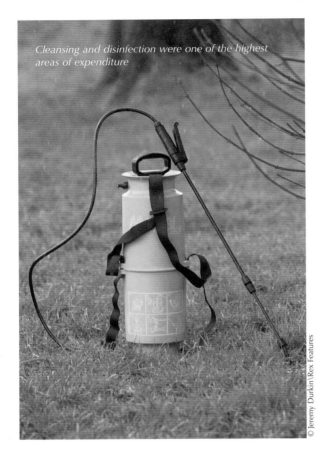

Cleansing and disinfection were one of the highest areas of expenditure

© Jeremy Durkin\Rex Features

could earn nearly three and a half times more in April 2001 than they could in February or March; and fees for temporary vets increased by 50 per cent between February and March 2001.

4.48 The Department's weak negotiating position resulted in it paying a high mark up for some of the land on which to build the mass burial pits. At Great Orton the land agent initially wanted to lease the land to the Department for 12 months at £10,000 an acre, ten times its value in normal market conditions. The Department negotiated the agent down to £6,000 an acre, six times its normal value. For the Ash Moor pit in Devon, the Department paid £350,000 for the land, which it estimated to be about three and half times the usual rate for such land.

Staff were stretched and some were inexperienced

4.49 There was intense pressure on procurement and other operational staff. At local Disease Control Centres slaughtermen, haulage contractors, heavy plant, machinery and materials had to be procured and deployed at dozens of farms in the area within a matter of days. The foot and mouth crisis required probably the biggest and broadest supply chain in Britain since the Second World War. After the first few days, there were shortages of administrative staff and managers to handle the increased volume of contract work and financial processing, both in local Disease Control Centres and at headquarters. New and often inexperienced staff were

58 A case study of cleansing and disinfecting

It is the Department's policy to pay for the cleansing and disinfecting of farms out of public funds.

Cleansing and disinfecting is necessary if farms are to be restocked with animals at an early stage. If cleansing and disinfecting does not take place, farms need to refrain from restocking for about 12 months. Article 11 of the Foot and Mouth Disease Order 1983 enables the Department to require the occupants of infected farms to cleanse and disinfect their own properties at their own expense or at the expense of the government. In most cases the Department chose to pay the costs of all cleansing and disinfecting from public funds as it considered that this was a priority measure of disease control. In 1967-68 poor cleansing and disinfecting had led to re-emergence of the disease.

At the start of the outbreak the Department envisaged that cleansing and disinfecting would normally be carried out by contractors. After the first few weeks, however, farmers were often given the first option to clean their own farms. The Department saw this as an opportunity to compensate some farmers and other agricultural workers affected by the disease.

By 24 May 2002 the Department had spent £295 million on cleansing and disinfecting, representing about 25 per cent of the amount paid in compensation to farmers for slaughtered animals. Around 40 per cent of the total expenditure on cleansing and disinfecting has been paid to farmers and 60 per cent to private contractors.

In the light of concerns about the escalating costs of cleansing and disinfecting work following advice from the Department, the Prime Minister called in July 2001 for an immediate review. The review - and subsequent investigations carried out by the Department - identified several cases where costs appeared to be excessive. In some cases the costs of cleansing and disinfecting far exceeded the value of the farmers' slaughtered animals. On one farm where the slaughtered livestock were valued at £4,000, cleansing and disinfecting had cost £59,000. At 13 farms in Gloucestershire the costs of cleansing and disinfecting were more than £100,000 for each farm.

The review concluded that:

- There were too few departmental staff to assess the work required for cleansing and disinfecting. Contractors and farmers were keen to increase the amount of work required and some supervisors were too ready to agree.

- Labour and plant hire rates were generous in some parts of the country and they encouraged contractors and farmers to inflate the amount of work done.

- Cleansing and disinfecting work started before financial budgets had been set. Lacking any clear expectation of what things would cost, the Department was not initially well placed to exercise effective financial control.

- In some areas the limited number of contractors capable of performing the work meant that the Department could not put the work out to competitive tender.

- Invoicing by some contractors and farmers was poor and this made it difficult for the Department to check the work carried out.

Analyses of the cost figures for cleansing and disinfecting show marked variations between Disease Control Centres. Compared with a national average of £36,000 per farm, average costs ranged from £25,000 in Exeter to £70,000 in Worcester. The Department told us that because of varying farming practices across the country, it would expect some variations in costs between one area and another.

Some of these variations were simply due to differences in the size of farms and the type of livestock carried. But there were also large variations in the rates paid for labour and the hire of equipment. For example, most of the work in Devon was carried out by farmers who were paid £10 an hour. In Worcester and Wales some contractors were paid up to £27.50 an hour.

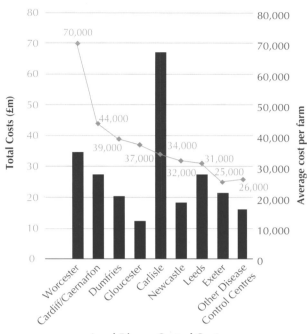

Average cost of cleansing and disinfecting by Disease Control Centre (up to October 2001)

■ Total costs (£m) ◆ Average cost per farm (£)

NOTE

These costs are at October 2001 and the Department is updating the figures. It expects that the update will lead to an increase in the average cost per farm. However, the figure for Cardiff/Caernarfon is expected to fall to around £38,000.

Source: Department for Environment, Food and Rural Affairs

Guidance on carrying out cleansing and disinfecting was complex and local Disease Control Centres adopted different practices where there were uncertainties, such as milking parlours and infected slurry. The cost of cleansing milking parlours, for example, varied from £650 to £10,000 depending on whether they were dismantled.

The National Farmers' Union told us that the tendering system for cleansing and disinfecting was poorly managed and that this made the system open to possible exploitation. At a local level, some contracts had been concluded in haste on the basis of incomplete cost estimates. Inadequate guidance had been issued to contractors as to how invoices should be presented, and on what costs could and could not be claimed for. Rates for items such as labour and plant hire appeared to vary from region to region.

Following the July 2001 review of cleansing and disinfecting costs, several new measures were introduced to improve value for money:

- Unsatisfactory contracts with contractors were terminated and others were renegotiated on more favourable terms to the Department. Contracts became fixed price and had to stipulate the cost to completion.

- Guidelines on cleansing standards were re-assessed and criteria laid down to avoid betterment of farm buildings and unnecessarily high cleansing standards.

- The Department reserved the right to withhold payment of all or part of the costs if cleansing was found to be unsatisfactory or work had been carried out unnecessarily. In these cases farmers would have to carry out cleansing at their own expense or not restock for 12 months.

brought in, some of whom were unfamiliar with the Department's systems, procedures and lines of accountability. Other more experienced staff were sometimes switched from procurement to carry out more urgent tasks, such as tracing infected animals and managing the deployment of veterinary staff. From the end of February 2001, local staff began to receive support and guidance from the Department's central procurement branches; and later some major contracts were awarded by the Joint Co-ordination Centre.

Some controls over purchasing were initially weak

4.50 From the start of the outbreak the Department activated its emergency purchasing arrangements to speed up procurement. These arrangements permitted local Disease Control Centres to award contracts whether oral or written without reference to the Department's headquarters branches and allowed paperwork to be prepared at a later date. Aspects of some contracts were initially agreed orally. Labour, materials and services were ordered by telephone, fax, or e-mail, without having to go through the Department's full procedures for authorisation and approval and the provision of supporting paperwork. When some contracts came to be written and formalised it was sometimes difficult for the parties involved to recall the detail of what had been agreed.

4.51 Controls were strained or did not always operate effectively:

- Many contracts which would normally be put out to tender were awarded without competition. By agreeing a price with just one contractor there was the risk it was not the lowest that could have been secured. In addition, the Department's weak negotiating position meant that some contractors were able to demand a premium for work related to foot and mouth disease.

- Often there were only a limited number of contractors both willing and able to handle the necessary tasks in the very limited time available. Contracts were therefore awarded to those companies that were available at the right time and place, such as those to Snowie Limited (**Figure 59**).

- Local contingency plans listed the names of approved firms who were expected to be able to supply the materials and services required. Approved firms would normally have to be vetted by the Department. However, because some local firms were unable to assist, or ran quickly out of supplies other firms and service providers had to be engaged without reference to the approved lists.

59 | **Snowie Limited**

Snowie Limited are a firm of waste management contractors based in Stirling, Scotland. During the outbreak they provided leak proof transport and disposal of thousands of animal carcasses in the North of England and Scotland and were involved in the construction and management of the mass burial site at Great Orton. To date they have received some £38 million from the Department. Their staff increased from 150 in February 2001 to 500 in April 2001 to cope with the demand for their services.

As with many other contractors engaged by the Department at the start of the outbreak in late February and early March 2001, the Department's initial contact with Snowie Limited was based on oral requests because of the necessary urgency. Snowie Limited were approached on 3 March 2001 by the Carlisle Disease Control Centre because staff at the Centre were aware that Snowie Limited had a fleet of leak proof lorries that were used under contract to transport meat and bonemeal from store to incineration and because of earlier contracts they had had with the Intervention Board Executive Agency (now the Rural Payments Agency). Snowie Limited responded positively to the request to assist.

From this early contact Snowie Limited's involvement in Cumbria expanded into all aspects of disposal, including transport, pyre burning, and burial of animals as the disease spread. Oral requests were later backed up with faxes, formally requesting the work to be carried out. On 4 April 2001 the Department's headquarters entered into a formal contract with Snowie Limited for the provision of plant, labour and materials for a three month period. The contract mainly involved collecting slaughtered animals from farms in Northern England and Scotland and work at the mass burial site in Great Orton. The work required at Great Orton was extensive and their contract was extended in June and again in September. In June the Department negotiated a reduction in Snowie Limited's costs.

As the peak of the disease passed and the Department gained additional resources to negotiate contracts, contracts were put out to tender involving competition in the normal way. Snowie Limited, for example, won some contracts against competition, such as the provision of plant, equipment and transport in Cumbria but lost others, for example, to treat and dispose of farm slurry and farm waste waters.

Snowie Limited's invoices were checked by forensic accountants and quantity surveyors employed by the Department and payments made to the company on a regular basis for worked carried out.

- Many contracts, some of which amounted to several million pounds, were agreed in a few hours when normally they might have taken weeks, if not months, to negotiate. In the early weeks of the outbreak some major contracts were awarded by Disease Control Centres without reference to expert procurement advisers.

■ In April 2001 a financial review was undertaken of the emergency purchasing procedures at Disease Control Centres. The review team found the procedures to be "cumbersome and inefficient"; and that there were no specific contracts for disposal and transport relating to emergency situations. Contracts with general terms and conditions therefore had to be used. In consequence, many contracts were agreed which provided for a notice period of 30 days. In some instances the Department was obliged to engage a firm for the whole period when there was insufficient work or curtail the contract early and risk a legal dispute. However, most contracts did not guarantee a minimum level of work and in these cases the Department was not obliged to pay contractors during notice periods.

Disputes with firms of contractors and service providers

4.52 A number of disputes have arisen between the Department and contractors about payment for work done. There have been three main areas of contention:

■ on quantum and accounting matters - for example, the rates paid for labour, transport and plant; payments made to subcontractors; rates for overnight accommodation and meals; and the fees paid to directors of companies;

■ on the interpretation of contracts; and

■ on the evidence provided to support invoices. The Department has been particularly concerned to ensure that contractors provide sufficient evidence of work carried out.

The Department is currently working to resolve these disputes and, whilst a few have been resolved to the satisfaction of both parties, many others have yet to be resolved.

4.53 The Department has employed forensic accountants to examine the invoices of 107 of the largest contractors, including the 86 companies awarded contracts worth more than £1 million. In total these 107 companies have submitted invoices worth £474 million and to date the Department has paid £402 million in respect of these claims (**Figure 60**). The Department is withholding payment of the remainder until it is satisfied that contractors have provided sufficient evidence of work carried out.

4.54 The Department's forensic accountants have completed their work on examining the invoices of 10 of the 107 companies. Five cases have been resolved amicably with the contractors concerned. On these cases the Department has negotiated a reduction of £3.7 million in the invoiced claims. The Department has stressed that these early cases should not be taken as an indication of the amounts the Department may save in relation to negotiations over other contractors' claims. Each case is being considered by the Department on its merits. In a further five completed cases the Department is in dispute with the contractors concerned about the amounts to be paid. Some of these cases are likely to result in legal proceedings.

4.55 In addition to the reductions to invoiced amounts, further savings have been generated through contract renegotiations and changes in invoicing practices as a result of work completed by the forensic accountants. A number of reductions have also been negotiated on accounts where investigation work is still in progress.

60 **Contractors' invoices examined by the forensic accountants employed by the Department**

	Number of Cases	Amounts invoiced by contractors	Amounts paid to date by the Department
		£m	£m
Forensic examination completed and amounts agreed with the contractor	5	51.6	47.3
Forensic examination completed and amounts in dispute	5	100.5	85.2
Forensic examination under way or yet to start	97	322.2	269.8
TOTAL	107	474.3	402.3

NOTE

All figures are estimates as at 23 May 2002 and are exclusive of VAT.

Source: The Department for Environment, Food and Rural Affairs

There were wide variations in the rates charged by contractors and others

4.56 The Department aimed to ensure that firms of contractors used reasonable rates for labour, materials, supplementary charges and plant given the scale of the outbreak and the need to eradicate the disease. It advised Disease Control Centres that they should base rates on those recommended by the Civil Engineering Contractors Association and the associated forms of contract. The Association's day rates were designed for emergency situations over a short period of time and were generally higher than the rates that would normally apply.

4.57 In practice Disease Control Centres based their negotiations with contractors on the Association's day rates, although there were variations to suit local circumstances. Many firms accepted the day rates as reasonable; others accepted lower rates. In areas such as Cumbria, where there was huge pressure on contractors to deliver work quickly, firms of contractors were initially able to negotiate much higher rates. Later in the crisis, when the demand for work had eased, the Department was able to negotiate much lower rates.

4.58 There were some wide variations in the rates charged by firms for carrying out similar tasks. For example, the Rural Payments Agency used commercial landfill sites as one method for disposing of carcasses under the livestock welfare scheme. Most landfill operating companies charged the Agency about £200 per tonne of carcass, exclusive of landfill tax. The Agency did not consider this good value but felt that it had little option as few operators wanted its business and the use of some well-located sites was imperative. Some operators charged the Agency about £300 a tonne, exclusive of landfill tax.

There was some wasted expenditure

4.59 Given the pressures under which the Department and other agencies were working it was perhaps inevitable that mistakes would be made and some unnecessary expenditure incurred. These problems need to be considered, however, in the context of the overall scale of the activities and the vast expenditure involved. Some of the problems were highly visible to those dealing directly with the Department, such as farmers and contractors, and received a lot of attention in the media. This did damage to the Department's reputation and made the task of eradicating the disease that much harder. Examples of these problems are shown in **Figure 61**.

61 Examples of problems experienced by the Department

In the early weeks of the crisis, the arrangements for the disposal and transportation of dead animals were often stretched and sometimes uncoordinated. A number of problems arose, including duplicate bookings, lorries turning up at the wrong farms, hire vehicles lying idle, drivers losing their way, and unsuitable lorries being hired from which waste products leaked on roads.

The allocation of tasks to Temporary Veterinary Inspectors by Disease Control Centres did not work well during the early weeks: bookings for farm inspections were duplicated and unnecessary journeys were made.

There were a number of procurement errors. For example, armed services personnel ordered 15 pneumatic stun guns by telephone from a firm in Kansas. The guns, which were required to kill sheep in a quicker and more efficient way, cost over £25,000. But it was found that the guns were not appropriate for slaughter at farms so they were never used and were put into storage until action could be taken to recover the £25,000 expenditure; a second order of 50 stun guns had to be cancelled. Efforts are underway to recover the £25,000 expenditure.

The Department took action to control costs

Specialist contract administrators were employed

4.60 From April 2001, the Department began to employ specialist contract administrators at each Disease Control Centre. Their main tasks were:

- to ensure that appropriate written contracts were in place;
- to negotiate better terms for the Department where they could;
- to encourage contractors to maintain accurate records of staff, materials and plant deployed;
- to monitor contractor performance, giving feedback to Departmental staff as necessary; and
- to provide expert advice to the Department.

4.61 Contract administration improved considerably and there were significant gains for the Department. In Carlisle, for example, new contracts for transportation of slaughtered animals were negotiated. In March 2001 the Department had paid £49 an hour for articulated lorries and £60 for eight-wheeled lorries, whether in use or on standby. Under new terms negotiated in May 2001, the Department paid £38 an hour for both types of vehicle and £28 an hour for vehicles on standby. The Department achieved a 50 per cent saving in the weekly cost of transport, from £800,000 a week in March 2001 to £400,000 a week in July 2001.

Quantity surveyors were employed

4.62 From March 2001 quantity surveyors were employed by the Department to give independent assurance that it was being charged reasonably for the work carried out by contractors. Quantity surveyors were tasked with agreeing schedules of rates for plant, equipment, materials and labour. They were also responsible for the validation and approval of contractors' invoices and checking that paperwork was correct. The Department employed up to 80 quantity surveyors at Disease Control Centres.

Dedicated teams of staff in Disease Control Centres improved the cost effectiveness of operations

4.63 The cost effectiveness of several functions improved when dedicated teams of staff ("cells") were set up at the Joint Co-ordination Centre and at Disease Control Centres. Armed services personnel provided expertise in management, planning and logistics. Separate cells were created to deal with infected premises, disposal, and cleansing and disinfecting. The disposal cell, for example, secured considerable improvements in the transport arrangements and the more economic disposal of carcasses and ash. For example, the rates charged by firms of contractors for the disposal of pyre ash fell from £163 a tonne to £96 a tonne as the disposal cell in London gained in experience.

The Department sought to recover value from surplus purchases

4.64 As the disease was brought under control, equipment and materials that had been used in its eradication were no longer needed. A considerable amount of office and other equipment also remained at Disease Control Centres. In May 2001 the Joint Co-ordination Centre commissioned a project to take stock of the levels of equipment and materials purchased by the Department and to realise the maximum value possible from any surpluses. By October 2001 Disease Control Centres had compiled inventories of most of their surplus equipment and materials.

4.65 The Department commissioned the Disposal Services Agency to dispose of surplus pyre material such as coal, railway sleepers and wood. Items of agricultural equipment and materials were also sold locally, some by auction. The Department expects to recover about £500,000 from these sales. The Department established a surplus stock register to enable surplus foot and mouth disease materials in an area where the disease was no longer active to be re-deployed to other areas still dealing with outbreaks. The Department and its Agencies have also re-deployed office, information technology and communications equipment that typically has a very low second-hand value, making substantial savings against the £6 million spent on this equipment. The Department estimates that to date £1.7 million has been saved by using the surplus stock register.

Financial controls over payments were strengthened after initial problems

4.66 Many of the Department's payment processes operated during the crisis as they would have done normally. The majority of farmers and firms of contractors received the compensation or payment amount that they were expecting after their animals were valued or work had been carried out. Though not designed to deal with such a major crisis, computer systems generally coped well with the huge volume of transactions. This was a significant achievement given the lack of preparation and demands placed on the systems.

Some financial controls were put under severe strain

4.67 In the first four months, the outbreak placed huge strains on a small but significant number of the Departments' systems of financial control, which resulted in their uneven implementation across local Disease Control Centres. The financial and communications systems of many suppliers and contractors were also at full stretch and this put further pressure on the Department's systems. Many firms of contractors doubled and trebled their workforce almost overnight, sometimes recruiting unskilled and untrained labour.

Information was often lacking to support the payment of bills

4.68 Controls were often put under strain because of a lack of evidence that could be verified and substantiated to support the payment of bills. With several thousand sites to supervise simultaneously, the Department was frequently unable to monitor the work being carried out by contractors, especially the slaughter and disposal of animals, and the cleansing and disinfecting of farms. Forensic accountants employed by the Department found that for over 40 per cent of contractors' invoices, the Department's officials and agents had not been able to confirm that the work claimed for had actually been carried out. The Department was very often unable to rely on timesheets and plant hire sheets provided by contractors.

4.69 The forensic accountants also found other omissions and errors:

- A lack of supporting documentation provided by contractors for travel expenses and claims for allowances.

- Time sheets for labour and plant use were not properly signed or authorised.

- Slaughterers did not always use the correct forms to record their activities and claim payment.

- It was not possible to verify from the documentation which plant and equipment was being used and which was being kept on "standby."

- Invoices contained a number of common errors. These included arithmetical mistakes, discrepancies between time worked and the availability of labour, overheads being charged to the Department which should have been borne by the contractor, and double charging.

Up to date information on current expenditure was not available at some Disease Control Centres

4.70 The Department collected information on expenditure related to the outbreak on a national basis both to brief Ministers and officials and for claims on the reserve, detailed supplementary estimates, policy decisions and business planning. Throughout the outbreak the Department's foot and mouth disease finance division issued a daily cost statement showing the estimated cost and actual expenditure of the operation. This was copied widely to Ministers, senior Departmental officials, the Treasury and the National Audit Office. However, information on actual expenditure or unit costs by local Disease Control Centres was not consistently available throughout the crisis and the quality of the information varied from one Centre to another. Without this information local finance managers were not always able to monitor expenditure or make comparisons between Disease Control Centres in order to identify good value for money practice. Some Centres set up their own computerised systems to track expenditure on certain activities, such as cleansing and disinfecting, but the systems were ad hoc and not necessarily based on consistent criteria across the country.

Qualification of audit opinion

4.71 The Comptroller and Auditor General qualified his audit opinion on the 2000-01 resource accounts of the Ministry of Agriculture, Fisheries and Food. This was partly because he was unable to obtain sufficient appropriate evidence to support sums included in the financial statements in respect of the handling and eradication of the outbreak of foot and mouth disease. There were weaknesses in controls over expenditure; particularly in the first four months of the response to the outbreak. As a result, at the time of the audit, the Ministry was unable to provide adequate evidence to support certain payments, in particular:

- Compensation payments: A Ministry official was present at the valuation of animals due to be culled and, with the farmer and the valuer, signed the valuation form. This form evidenced the amount of compensation that should be paid. In many cases

slaughter took place immediately following valuation but in other cases there was a delay. The Ministry's policy was for subsequent slaughter to be under supervision by Ministry officials or their agents. For a significant number of compensation payments there was no documentary evidence of slaughter. However, the Department told us that there is no evidence to suggest that any animals which were valued and on which compensation was paid were not subsequently slaughtered.

The Ministry's database for compensation payments did not reconcile with the numbers of animals slaughtered according to the Disease Control System. The two databases were based on different records. The Department has undertaken a substantial exercise to reconcile the two databases and expects to complete the exercise by May 2002. At the time of the Comptroller and Auditor General's audit the reconciliation was only 75 per cent complete. By mid May 2002 it was 95 per cent complete.

- Non-compensation payments. There was insufficient evidence to support invoices from contractors for hours worked. And initially weak controls over the monitoring of cleansing and disinfecting work meant that there was a risk of inappropriately high payments being made. The Department is in serious commercial dispute with a range of contractors and formal litigation is underway in a number of cases (see paragraph 4.52 above).

In addition the Ministry was unable to provide sufficient evidence that the provision for costs included in the accounts represented a reliable estimate of total expenditure.

The scale of the activity and the enormous task involved opened financial systems to the risk of fraud and abuse

Investigations by the Department of alleged frauds

4.72 The financial control weaknesses referred to above would have made the Department more exposed to the risk of fraud and abuse. In June 2001 the Department issued guidance to staff at Disease Control Centres on how they should deal with allegations of fraud. The guidance required staff receiving allegations of fraud to establish as much information as they could about the dates, time and place of the alleged events. Staff were required to assess whether there was substance to the allegations by researching the names of those involved and the existence of any places specified. Allegations which appeared to have some basis for believing fraud may have been committed were referred to regional managers. On the basis of the evidence regional managers decided whether the information warranted further investigation. If cases did require further investigation, they were referred to the Department's Investigation Branch in London, where the Chief Investigation Officer would determine whether a criminal investigation should be undertaken. Any allegations of fraud involving Departmental staff were to be reported first to personnel units at regional offices and then referred to the Chief Investigation Officer if appropriate.

4.73 The Department received many calls from members of the public who made allegations which were not specific or based on hearsay. For example, there were many allegations made over the telephone that "contractors were committing fraud". In addition there were articles in the press and other sources which made general allegations. The Department told us that all substantive allegations received were pursued.

4.74 By mid May 2002 the Investigation Branch had received 33 substantive allegations of fraud or abuse connected with foot and mouth disease (**Figure 62**). These allegations were received from members of staff, farmers and members of the public. Of the 33 allegations received: 3 cases are being prosecuted; 16 cases are still under investigation, of which 4 are with lawyers to determine whether prosecution would be appropriate; and 14 cases have been closed, either because the allegations were found to be unproven after investigation, or because there was insufficient evidence to warrant a prosecution, or because there were satisfactory explanations for the events that occurred.

4.75 The Department's Investigation Branch examined the evidence available on 4 cases where it was alleged that people had deliberately infected animals. In 3 cases the

investigators considered that the only evidence was based on hearsay and the cases were not pursued. The other case involved a farmer alleged to have deliberately infected stock he had recently purchased in order to claim compensation on the animals. The case file was passed to the Department's lawyers for possible prosecution but they considered that there was insufficient evidence to prove that the farmer had deliberately infected his animals and the case was dropped.

4.76 Eleven of the cases under investigation concern allegations relating to claims for cleansing and disinfecting work. The nature of the allegations is varied. They involve the exaggeration of hours worked by contractors, inflated claims, claims about work undertaken that had not been carried out, and claims made by workmen who were working elsewhere or were on holiday.

4.77 The four cases under investigation regarding compensation claims concern:

■ an allegation that the estimate for work to remedy damage caused by cleansing and disinfection has been exaggerated by a contractor;

■ an allegation that compensation has been paid on the basis of false claims in respect of the pedigree status of some of a farmer's animals;

■ an allegation that a farmer claimed compensation for an exaggerated number of hens destroyed during the outbreak; and

62 | **Allegations of fraud concerning foot and mouth disease**

Type of allegation received by the Department	Number of allegations received	Outcome of investigation		
		Case closed, no further action	Prosecuted/to be prosecuted	Under investigation
People deliberately infecting animals	4	4	0	0
False claims for cleansing and disinfecting work	17	6	0	11
False claims for compensation for slaughtered animals or other items destroyed.	8	3	1	4
Frauds or abuse by Departmental staff	3 (see note)	1	2	0
Other false claims for payment	1	0	0	1
TOTAL	**33**	**14**	**3**	**16**

NOTE

One of the three cases relates to 18 people.

Source: The Department for Environment, Food and Rural Affairs, as at 17 May 2002.

■ an allegation of collusion between valuers and a farmer to inflate the value of the farmer's animals.

In addition, prosecution has been initiated in respect of a claim for compensation of £3,652 for bales of straw destroyed. The claim has not been paid.

4.78 The Department received allegations of criminal activity involving 20 of its employees. Eighteen of these people worked at the Exeter Disease Control Centre and were suspended on full pay whilst the Department investigated claims for hotel expenses. Of the 18 staff members, 3 are to be prosecuted and 15 are to be the subject of internal disciplinary proceedings. A member of staff from the Leeds Disease Control Centre is being prosecuted for irregularities concerning false overtime and travel claims. One other staff investigation has been closed.

Investigations by the Rural Payments Agency of alleged frauds

4.79 The Counter Fraud and Compliance Unit of the Rural Payments Agency investigated allegations of fraud made about the Livestock Welfare (Disposal) Scheme. Some 124 allegations were received by the Rural Payments Agency in respect of this Scheme. The allegations concerned farmers who made claims for payment under the Scheme on unfounded welfare reasons or who incorrectly classified their animals so that they could claim a higher payment than that to which they were entitled, for example, claiming sheep were pregnant when they were not. Of the 124 allegations made, there was insufficient evidence to warrant an investigation by the Counter Fraud and Compliance Unit in 78. The Unit investigated the other 46 cases and found insufficient evidence in 40 cases to support the allegations. Most of the allegations involved animals that had been slaughtered and destroyed and there was no way of gathering sufficient evidence to substantiate the allegations.

4.80 Three investigations were concluded which have led the Agency to withhold monies or to seek recovery of payments from farmers:

■ A farmer made a claim for payment for 56 sheep which had died or been slaughtered prior to his claim. A payment of £4,536 was withheld.

■ A farmer claimed for more sheep than were slaughtered under the scheme. The Agency is seeking to recover £59,373.

■ A farmer incorrectly classified his ewes and lambs. The Agency is seeking to recover £2,421.

The remaining three investigations are on-going.

There were delays in making payments to farmers, contractors and others

Farmers

4.81 The Department aimed to pay farmers' claims under the slaughter scheme within two to three weeks of receiving notification of the value of their animals. This target proved impossible to meet, however, as staff were swamped by the volume of claims, which needed to be properly checked. For the early cases there were delays in some payments of six to eight weeks, although some were paid quickly. When the number of claims peaked in early May 2001, some payments were being delayed by up to 6 to 8 weeks. The National Farmers' Union told us that the delays caused real financial hardship to some farmers. The time taken to pay farmers was the subject of many complaints to the Department.

4.82 During May 2001 over 100 staff were recruited to process payments. The Department set up 15 helplines for farmers who could also contact their local Disease Control Centres or the Department's headquarters. The Department followed up enquiries on late payment and cases of hardship. Farmers were informed about when they could expect payment wherever possible and the backlog of claims was cleared by the end of May 2001. From June 2001 the Department adopted a target to pay farmers within 21 days, and this was met in almost every case.

4.83 For the Livestock Welfare (Disposal) Scheme, the Rural Payments Agency set a target to pay claims within 21 days of the date of slaughter. The Agency was unable to meet this target: by 19 July 2001 only two per cent of some 4,500 approved claims had been paid within 21 days. The average payment time was 48 days; and around 18 per cent of claims were paid 60 or more days after slaughter. The delays were caused by the huge volume of applications and the amount of checking required on each claim. The speed of payment gradually improved as the Agency allocated more staff to the task. By mid-August 2001 the backlog in claims had been largely removed and most payments were being made within 28 days of slaughter.

Contractors

4.84 The Department sought to pay contractors within 30 days of receipt and agreement of invoices. But a huge backlog of unpaid invoices built up in Disease Control Centres and some contractors experienced long delays in receiving their money. The problem was particularly acute in the first two months. At Carlisle, for example, over 1,000 invoices dating back to late February had not been paid by the second week in April. Several large

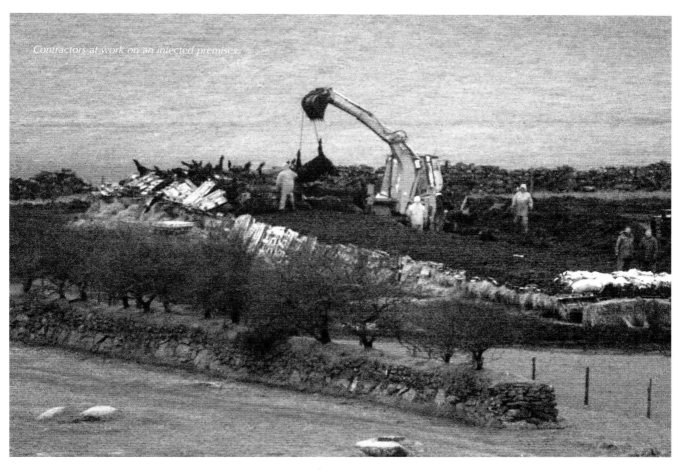

Contractors at work on an infected premises.

contractors claimed that for a brief period they had been "bankrolling" the crisis. Some private contractors ran into serious cash flow problems. Some contractors took several months to submit invoices to the Department because their own systems became overwhelmed.

4.85 The time taken to pay bills gradually improved and the 30 day payment target was eventually met. Between 1 April and 30 September 2001 the Department received over 90,000 invoices, of which 82 per cent were paid within 30 days of receipt. In total some 235,000 invoices were processed by the end of April 2002. In some cases payments on account have been made where agreeing final accounts has been delayed because of the need to verify the amounts claimed.

Temporary Veterinary Inspectors

4.86 There were particular difficulties with the terms and conditions of Temporary Veterinary Inspectors. Difficulties arose because of the very large numbers that had to be appointed in a very short space of time. The difficulties led to payment delays, errors in pay and numerous complaints and disputes. The Department had provided guidance to Disease Control Centres on the inspectors' terms and conditions of employment. This was incomplete, however, and gave rise to confusion about the fees payable to inspectors "on call" but not working, annual leave entitlements, tax

deductions, and the rates of pay for travel and overnight accommodation. These issues were addressed and revised guidance was issued. Further work is continuing on a revision to the procedure for the appointment of these staff.

The Department took action to improve financial controls

A dedicated Finance Unit was set up

4.87 On 23 April 2001 the Joint Co-ordination Centre set up a specialist Finance Unit for foot and mouth disease at the Department's headquarters. The Deputy Head of Internal Audit was appointed as the Head of the Unit because of his familiarity with financial control issues. Other members of Internal Audit were seconded to the Unit for two months to establish its structure and responsibilities.

4.88 A member of the Unit was assigned to improve the financial and accounting controls in Disease Control Centres. He visited each Disease Control Centre to assess the level of compliance with procedures and controls and his findings and recommendations were acted upon. The Unit also recruited experienced finance staff and placed them in key posts at headquarters and the Disease Control Centres. This was an immense task:

at the height of the crisis, the Department used 220 financial staff on foot and mouth work.

4.89 A Financial Control Team was set up to ensure that financial controls at Disease Control Centres were consistent with each other. The team had the responsibility to visit Centres, to provide assistance on financial procedures, and to report back to headquarters on the Centres' compliance with procedures and the provision of financial information. Monthly meetings of finance managers were held to improve communications between Disease Control Centres and to promote good practice.

Financial responsibilities were reorganised

4.90 On 1 May 2001 financial responsibility for foot and mouth disease expenditure was brought together under the Head of Foot and Mouth Operations in the Joint Co-ordination Centre in London. Day to day financial responsibility was delegated to the Regional Operations Directors appointed to Disease Control Centres. These arrangements relieved vets of involvement in financial matters, established clearer lines of responsibility, and improved financial control. Regional Operations Directors were made responsible for approving foot and mouth expenditure, authorising payments, providing financial information and seeking to ensure that value for money was achieved. Divisional Veterinary Managers were made responsible for advising on expenditure for disease control purposes.

A team of forensic accountants was employed to check invoices

4.91 The Department employed a team of forensic accountants from April 2001 to assist in the checking of contractors' invoices and to advise the Department as to how much contractors should be paid. Up to 15 forensic accountants were posted to the Disease Control Centres to examine the invoices of all contractors who claimed to have carried out more than £1 million worth of work. By May 2002 the forensic accountants had carried out investigations and examined invoices totalling more than £330 million (excluding VAT), including the invoices of 45 of the largest firms of contractors.

4.92 The Department is calculating how much money has been saved through the work of quantity surveyors, forensic accountants, claim surveyors and contract managers. Initial estimates are that the quantity surveyors and contract managers alone have saved the Department £16.8 million.

Hire charges were monitored

4.93 Systems were set up at each Disease Control Centre to monitor the quantity and cost of goods on hire (heavy plant and equipment, cars, mobile phones and office equipment). This led to reductions in the amount of goods on hire and as a result, by March 2002, some £1.2 million had been saved.

Glossary

Biosecurity	The precautions taken to minimise the risk that the virus might be spread inadvertently by those working with livestock and visiting farms, and after infected animals have been slaughtered and disposed of. These include thorough cleansing and disinfecting of the person, equipment and vehicles by those working on and visiting farms, minimising inessential contact with susceptible animals and cleansing and disinfecting of premises where animals that had been infected or exposed were present.
Cabinet Office Briefing Room	Inter-departmental body, activated on 22 March 2001, to oversee, monitor and direct the operational efforts to eradicate the disease.
Contiguous Premises	A category of dangerous contacts where susceptible livestock are believed to have been exposed to infection because of their proximity to a neighbouring infected premises.
Controlled Area	The area affected by general control on movement of susceptible animals.
Dangerous Contacts	Premises where it is believed that animals have been exposed to foot and mouth disease infection by virtue of a known contact with infected animals or by contact through movements of vehicles, persons or things believed to be contaminated with virus.
Departmental Emergency Control Centre	The national emergency control centre set up, on 21 February 2001, at the State Veterinary Services' Page Street headquarters.
Disease Control Centre	A centre set up, normally at the Animal Health Divisional Office, to oversee disease control operations within an Animal Health Division.
Disease Control System	The core database used during the 2001 epidemic containing information on infected and other premises, restrictions served and actions taken.
Infected Area	An area of a minimum of 10 kilometres around an infected premises in which strict movement and biosecurity restrictions are in force.
Infected Premises	A farm, or other location with livestock, where foot and mouth disease has been confirmed on the basis of clinical findings by a veterinary surgeon or positive laboratory tests.
Joint Co-ordination Centre (JCC)	Body set up, on 26 March 2001, at the Department's Page Street headquarters to co-ordinate disease control operations across the country and Departmental input into operational policy.
Protection Zone	The area within a three kilometre boundary of infected premises.
Regional Operations Directors	Senior Civil Servants who, from 19 March 2001, were sent to certain Disease Control Centres to manage non-veterinary activities, such as slaughter and disposal, and organise the administrative input.
Restricted Infected Area	Area of tight biosecurity provisions governing movement of vehicles, public cleansing and disinfecting stations and increased enforcement activity.

Serology

The scientific study of blood serum.

Slaughter on Suspicion premises

Premises where on veterinary examination there are insufficient grounds to confirm disease but where there are clinical signs that cannot exclude the possibility of disease being present. Animals are culled and samples taken to confirm the presence/absence of disease. Cases giving positive results, or those that are subsequently confirmed on clinical grounds, are classified as infected premises.

Surveillance Zone

The area lying between three and 10 kilometres of infected premises.

Appendix 1

Foot and Mouth Disease Outbreak: Chronology of Events 2001 - 2002

Date	Cumulative Cases	Action
19 February 2001	0	Meat Hygiene Service vet at Cheale Meats abattoir reports suspected Foot and Mouth Disease in 27 sows. Samples sent to the Institute for Animal Health at Pirbright. Forms A and C issued prohibiting livestock movements within eight kilometres of the infected premises.
20 February	1	Samples test positive for type O Foot and Mouth Disease virus. First case confirmed in evening. European Commission informed of outbreak; it in turn notifies other Member States. Department of Health and Food Standards Agency confirm no implications for human health or food. Ministry of Agriculture, Fisheries and Food establish Foot and Mouth Disease website. Ministry of Agriculture, Fisheries and Food warns Ministry of Defence of possibility of future request for military assistance.
21 February	2	Infected Area round the first infected premises declared and animal movements within it banned. Ban on moving animals susceptible to foot and mouth disease and non-treated products from the entire UK imposed by European Commission. Baroness Hayman makes a statement on the outbreak in the House of Lords (House of Commons in recess). The statement also confirms no implications for human health via the food chain. National Disease Emergency Control Centre established at Ministry Headquarters in Page Street.
22 February	3	Ministry issues advice to farmers to operate to high hygiene standards and to the public to reduce contact with livestock and farms.
23 February	6	Heddon-on-the Wall case in Northumberland - first outside Essex. Great Britain is made a Controlled Area from 5pm with immediate standstill on all foot and mouth disease susceptible animal movements until 2 March; fairs and markets closed and deer and fox hunting and hare coursing prohibited. Ministry halts Common Agricultural Policy subsidy inspections for biosecurity reasons. First national stakeholders meeting of a regular series held in London with Ministers and officials. Department for Culture, Media and Sport alerts rural tourism trade associations to Ministry advice issued on 22 February. Public Health Laboratory Service issues factsheet on human health, confirming risks very small and human cases very rare.
25 February	7	First case in Devon confirmed. Environment Agency National Incident Room opened to co-ordinate Agency response. Environment Agency and the Ministry of Agriculture, Fisheries and Food issue joint statement confirming that the Agency regards disposal of carcasses as an emergency situation, under the terms of the Environmental Protection Act 1990 and Waste Management Licensing Regulations 1994.
27 February	16	First confirmed cases in Wales (Anglesey). Local authorities given right to close footpaths and rights of way outside Infected Areas. Invitation to Scottish Executive Rural Affairs Department and National Assembly for Wales Agriculture Department to locate representatives in Page Street.

Date	Cumulative Cases	Action
28 February	24	First confirmed case in Cumbria.
1 March	31	First confirmed case in Dumfries and Galloway. Countryside Agency estimates foot and mouth disease implications for rural businesses - potential £2 billion loss. Formal notification to Ministry of Defence that the Ministry of Agriculture, Fisheries and Food might seek military assistance.
2 March	38	Great Britain continues as a Controlled Area. Movement to approved slaughterhouses of animals intended for the human food chain allowed to resume under licence. Restrictions on drivers' hours relaxed for hauliers of agricultural products/supplies because of the need to undertake foot and mouth disease precautions. First vets arrive to reinforce operations from outside the UK (from the Republic of Ireland).
3 March	48	Minister of Agriculture announces a major review of safeguards to cut risks of future animal disease outbreaks.
5 March	75	Department for Culture, Media and Sport issues guidance on 'Visiting the Countryside for Tourism, Sport or Recreation'.
6 March	80	EU Standing Veterinary Committee maintains the measures in place in relation to UK. Environment Agency announces disposal hierarchy, taking environmental issues into account. This places rendering and incineration first. Ministry issues advisory leaflets on animal welfare problems to farmers and farming organisations. Ministers meet at annual Tourism Summit to review impact of foot and mouth disease. Guidance issued to local authorities on use of footpath closure powers and placed on Ministry website. Agreement with Central Association of Agricultural Valuers on payment to valuers for valuing livestock during the outbreak.
9 March	126	Occupational Licences and Local Movement Licences introduced to allow animal movements for welfare reasons. Minister of State (Ministry of Agriculture, Fisheries and Food) writes to the Minister of State (Ministry of Defence) to seek support from Royal Army Veterinary Corps and assistance from military personnel for slaughter in particular circumstances.
13 March	199	Case in France reported to the European Commission. Prime Minister chairs a meeting on the wider impact of foot and mouth disease with representatives of rural business and other countryside bodies.
14 March	219	Rural Task Force - 1st meeting chaired by Minister of Environment. Further meetings at weekly and then fortnightly intervals. Royal Army Veterinary Corps deploys four vets. Meeting between Ministry of Agriculture, Fisheries and Food and Ministry of Defence agrees deployment of armed forces for logistic and organisational purposes. Director of Foot and Mouth Disease Operations appointed.
15 March	250	Minister of Agriculture in statement to Parliament explains policy of culling sheep within 3km of infected premises in part of Cumbria; intensive patrolling in Devon and continued programme of tracing and slaughter of dangerous contacts across country; and announces new welfare movement schemes.

Date	Cumulative Cases	Action
16 March	270	Long Distance Welfare Movement Scheme starts. Power for local authorities to impose large-scale footpath closures revoked. Department for the Environment, Transport and the Regions issues guidance on visiting the countryside. Launch of Countryside Agency website linked to local authority rights of way information.
19 March	352	First Regional Operations Directors appointed in Cumbria and Devon to strengthen Disease Control Centres and support veterinary effort. Others appointed over following two weeks. Military Commanders appointed for these regions and military deployment followed in other regions.
20 March	394	Prime Minister initiates daily interdepartmental meetings, chaired by Ministry of Agriculture, Fisheries and Food Ministers to co-ordinate and drive forward action to control of the disease.
21 March	437	Minister of Agriculture announces in Parliament action taken to speed response: allowing vets on the ground to slaughter without waiting for a decision from vets in Page Street and introducing a standard valuation tariff to reduce delays in starting slaughter. Presentation by the epidemiologists of their models. The groups attending this meeting later formed the core of the Chief Scientific Adviser's Science Group. First cull of foot and mouth disease affected animals in the Netherlands.
22 March	479	Cabinet Office Briefing Room opens. 'Visiting the Countryside - how you can help' advert in the national press. First formal veterinary risk assessment of risk that walkers could spread the disease published. Flat-rate standard valuation system introduced for animals slaughtered as part of disease eradication, with farmers retaining the right to opt for specific valuations by valuers. Livestock Welfare (Disposal) Scheme launched.
23 March	514	First epidemiological forecasts presented by teams from Imperial College and Edinburgh University. On the basis of the forecast, the Chief Scientific Adviser proposed the 24 hour infected premises/48 hour contiguous cull policy in the Cabinet Office Briefing Room at its first meeting chaired by the Prime Minister. Sheep within 3km of infected premises in the Carlisle/Solway area to be slaughtered. 101 Logistic Brigade HQ deployed in the Ministry's headquarters in London (Page Street).
24 March	577	The Chief Scientists' Group is formed.
26 March	644	Great Orton mass burial site receives first carcasses. Joint Co-ordination Centre established in Page Street. Foot and Mouth Disease Science Group starts daily meetings, most chaired by Chief Scientific Adviser.
27 March	692	Minister of Agriculture's Parliamentary statement confirms 24hr/48hr slaughter targets; announces consultations on banning pigswill and 20-day movement restrictions, simplified valuation arrangements, commitment to seek Standing Veterinary Committee's contingent approval for vaccination, consideration to be given to methods for controlling illegal meat imports; and a future review of operation of the livestock sector. Meeting between Imperial and Cambridge teams to compare output of their two epidemiological models.
28 March	741	Guidance and News Release on access to the countryside, including a code for walkers. Department for Culture, Media and Sport issues guidance to tourist attractions to help them open or re-open.
29 March	779	Vaccination seminar held at 10 Downing Street attended by Prime Minister, Minister of Agriculture, Chief Veterinary Officer, Chief Scientific Adviser, Government and non-Government scientists.

appendix one

Date	Cumulative Cases	Action
30 March	829	Largest number of cases (50) reported in a day. Slaughtering started under Livestock Welfare (Disposal) Scheme. Ministry formally requests European Commission to reserve 5.5m doses of vaccine. Contingent use of vaccination authorised under Commission Decision. Spongiform Encephalopathy Advisory Committee meets to consider BSE aspects of various disposal options for cattle carcasses.
31 March	874	Joint Co-ordination Committee advises Regional Operations Directors of Spongiform Encephalopathy Advisory Committee advice, with agreement from the Environment Agency, that cattle born before 1 August 1996 must be rendered or burned, and that those born after 1 August 1996 could be buried in mass burial sites but not licensed commercial landfill sites.
1 April	909	Prime Minister launches campaign to assure tourists that Britain is 'Open for Business'.
2 April	946	Prime Minister announces a delay in local elections until 7 June.
3 April	990	Minister of Agriculture meets leaders of the dairy and food industries to discuss the implications of vaccinating cattle on meat and milk supplies.
4 April	1024	Department for the Environment, Transport and the Regions writes to Chief Executives of Local Authorities providing details of the foot and mouth 'Disposal Hierarchy' and a list of suitable landfill sites for the disposal of Livestock Welfare (Disposal) Scheme carcasses and the possible disposal of sheep and pigs from contiguous cull premises (but not from disease infected premises).
6 April	1083	Ministry announces new livestock movement licences (local movement and longer distance).
8 April	1134	Minister of Agriculture writes to 85,000 livestock farmers providing advice on biosecurity, encouraging continued co-operation with present slaughter policy and urging them not to move animals without a licence.
9 April	1163	Minister of Agriculture's Parliamentary statement confirms 24 hour target for culling susceptible animals on infected premises and 48 hour target for susceptible animals on contiguous premises; explains that payments to farmers of optional agrimonetary compensation would be made that week; notes that the position on vaccination was being kept under review; and refers to the possibility of releasing some areas from restrictions.
15 April	1320	14% of footpaths open.
18 April	1382	Government states vaccination in North Cumbria and Devon under consideration but listening to views of farmers and food industry. Chief Veterinary Officer and Chief Scientific Adviser explain limited vaccination proposals to media and stakeholders. National Farmers' Union still not convinced of the argument for vaccination. 500,000 doses of vaccine from EU vaccine bank confirmed as immediately available as a contingency measure. Chief Scientific Adviser and Science Group meet National Farmers' Union (and again on 19 April) to discuss vaccination.
19 April	1397	First lifting of Infected Areas, affecting Northamptonshire, Milton Keynes, Leicestershire, Lincolnshire, Nottinghamshire and Rutland.
20 April	1412	Letter to livestock farmers with information on vaccination.

Date	Cumulative Cases	Action
24 April	1461	Department of Health issues 'Guidance on Measures to Minimise Risk to Public Health from the Slaughter and Disposal of Animals', including hierarchy of disposal options and advice on the location and use of pyres, and also 'Foot and Mouth - Effects on Health of Emissions from Pyres used for the Disposal of Animals'.
25 April	1479	Environment Department minister Beverley Hughes launches Countryside Agency grant scheme to assist local authorities to adopt a consistent risk-based approach to re-opening rights of way and access land. Ministry of Agriculture, Fisheries and Food and Department for the Environment, Transport and the Regions issue revised guidance on re-opening rights of way.
26 April	1482	Minister of Agriculture's Parliamentary statement refines policy on the contiguous cull to give local veterinary discretion over culling of cattle if adequate biosecurity, and proposes new arrangements for rare breeds and hefted sheep; explains that the use of vaccination was now less likely; announces the revision of the Livestock Welfare Disposal Scheme rates from 30 April and outlines the Government's intentions to identify ways of assisting the recovery of the farming sector.
30 April	1518	Minister of Agriculture's letter to all livestock farmers explains the modifications to the contiguous cull policy.
3 May	1543	Minister of Agriculture announces a ban from 24 May on swill feeding livestock.
7 May	1563	Last carcasses into Great Orton mass burial site. No pyres lit in England and Wales after this date. Backlog of animals awaiting disposal eliminated.
17 May	1603	26% of footpaths open.
23 May	1633	Revised guidance to local authorities on re-opening of rights of way in light of new Veterinary Risk Assessment on the risks of path users spreading disease. Movement of animals from premises under Form D restrictions allowed.
24 May	1635	Ban on the swill feeding of catering waste to livestock comes into effect. Replacement of the slaughter policy by serological testing in the 3 km protection zones in Cumbria. Special Spongiform Encepalopathy Advisory Committee Working Group advises on potential risks from cattle over five years old that were already buried; the relative risks of methods for disposal of pyre ash; use of feed lorries for transportation of carcasses.
28 May	1657	Chief Veterinary Officer and Chief Scientific Adviser issue joint statement on Settle outbreak stressing the importance of biosecurity.
31 May	1672	Department of Health publishes a risk assessment of carcass disposal options available during the outbreak and also announces a public health monitoring programme in relation to the disposal of animal carcasses during the outbreak.
8 June	1714	Prime Minister announces the creation of a new 'Department for Environment, Food and Rural Affairs'.
14 June	1740	Secretary of State for Environment, Food and Rural Affairs stresses the need for continued effort to be focussed on the complete eradication of the disease and states that mass burial sites are national assets. 55% of footpaths open.
22 June	1773	Department for Environment, Food and Rural Affairs announces intention to revoke most local authority footpath closures.

Date	Cumulative Cases	Action
4 July	1807	Government's public information campaign on biosecurity launched.
6 July	1814	Biosecurity video and leaflet sent to all livestock farmers, stakeholders and vets.
20 July	1869	Revocation from midnight of many of the remaining local authority closures of public rights of way. Countryside Agency launches publicity campaign around newly revised access code welcoming people to the countryside and advising on ways of avoiding spreading foot and mouth disease.
23 July	1880	Review of costs of cleansing and disinfecting announced with the aim of ensuring value for money, following concerns over size and quality of invoices.
27 July	1895	85% of footpaths open.
29 July	1898	Restricted Infected Area declared around Thirsk, to deal with a cluster of new cases. It introduces tight biosecurity provisions governing movement of vehicles, public cleansing and disinfecting stations and increased enforcement activity.
30 July	1902	Option of valuation at standard rates removed.
3 August	1922	Cleansing and disinfecting restarts with stricter rules.
7 August	1927	Restricted Infected Area declared in the Penrith Spur.
9 August	1937	Announcement of Government Inquiries - Policy Commission into Food and Farming, Royal Society and Lessons Learned. 90% of footpaths open.
26 August	1975	Restricted Infected Area declared around Allendale and Hexham, to deal with a cluster of new cases.
28 August	1985	Announcement of Autumn movement arrangements starting from 17 September. Introduces county basis for categorising disease risk; confirms no cattle or sheep markets and sets out licensing system for moving animals.
3 September	1996	Light Lambs Scheme introduced extending the Livestock Welfare (Disposal) Scheme to deal with lambs unable to find a market.
30 September	2026	Last confirmed case of foot and mouth disease.
18 October	2026	Lord Haskins' Report on Rural Recovery after Foot and Mouth Disease published. Rural Task Force Report on Tackling Impact of Foot and Mouth on Rural Economy published.
22 October	2026	Standing Veterinary Committee permits exports of pigmeat from counties which have not had a case of foot and mouth disease in this outbreak and which are not adjoining high risk counties.
31 October	2026	Animal Health (Amendment) Bill published. Proposes greater powers to slaughter any animals where necessary to prevent the spread of disease, adjusted arrangements for compensation and strengthened enforcement powers.
28 November	2026	Last foot and mouth disease Infected Area covering parts of Cumbria, North Yorkshire and County Durham lifted at midnight.

Date	Cumulative Cases	Action
7 December	2026	Guidance to local authorities on re-opening rights of way allowing paths across fields of premises under restriction to be re-opened.
17 December	2026	Hunting with dogs allowed to resume in disease-free counties subject to a temporary system of disease control permits. Livestock Welfare (Disposal) Scheme ends.
1 January 2002	2026	Counties of Cumbria, Durham, and North Yorkshire declared free of foot and mouth for animal movement purposes, following huge surveillance operation.
14 January	2026	Northumberland, the last county, declared free of foot and mouth disease for animal movement purposes.
16 January	2026	EU Standing Veterinary Committee lifts restrictions on exports of British meat, animal products and livestock. Exports of live sheep still banned, but exports of live pigs, fresh meat and meat products permitted.
22 January	2026	UK regains international foot and mouth disease free status at meeting of Office Internationale des Epizooties (OIE). Clears way for UK to resume trade in animals and animal products with member countries of OIE.
11 February	2026	Foot and Mouth Disease Controlled Area lifted in England and Wales (Scotland 18 February). Animal movement controls eased and some livestock markets permitted to re-open under the Interim Regime.
1 March	2026	99.5% of all footpaths open

Appendix 2

Comparison with the 1967-68 outbreak

Between 1954 and 1967, isolated outbreaks of foot and mouth disease in the United Kingdom had occurred almost every year. Consequently, at the time of the last major outbreak in 1967-68, there was much greater awareness of the disease. Some of the key differences between the 1967-68 and 2001 epidemics are shown in the following table:

	1967-68 epidemic	2001 epidemic
Date the first case was confirmed	25 October 1967, at Bryn Farm in Shropshire.	20 February 2001, at an abattoir in Essex.
Date the last case was diagnosed	4 June 1968	30 September 2001.
Length of epidemic	222 days	221 days
Speed of idenficiation of the source case	Reported to the Department's vet within four days of the onset of clinical signs.	Reported to the Department's vets around three weeks after the likely onset of clinical signs.
Extent of initial 'seeding'	There were up to 24 almost simultaneous primary outbreaks deriving from a consignment of infected frozen lamb carcasses from Argentina distributed in Cheshire and Shropshire. This led to an early explosion in cases, with 490 cases occurring during one week in mid-November 1967.	There was one source case, but its identification, three weeks after infection, meant the disease had been spread around the country as a result of movements of, mainly, sheep through markets and dealers. At least 57 premises, in nine geographical groups, are now known to have been 'seeded' with infection by 20 February 2001. Each case would be likely to give rise to further cases because of the infectious nature of the virus with the result that the outbreak would be extremely large.
The extent to which the disease spread throughout the United Kingdom (Figure A1)	The disease was mainly concentrated in the Cheshire Plain, affecting in particular dairying areas of Cheshire, Staffordshire, Montgomeryshire, Denbighshire, Shropshire and Flintshire. There were outbreaks in 16 counties.	The disease was widespread and affected 44 British counties, unitary authorities and metropolitan districts from the Scottish Borders in the north, to Anglesey in the west, and to Cornwall in the far south west. There were concentrations of infection in Cumbria, Devon, Dumfries and Galloway, Northumberland and North Yorkshire.
Overall number of 'infected premises' (Figure A2	2,364 The peak of the epidemic was higher and earlier than in 2001 because of the large number of simultaneous primary outbreaks.	2,026
Number of animals slaughtered for disease control purposes	442,000 (49 per cent cattle, 26 per cent pigs and 25 per cent sheep).	More than four million (85 per cent sheep, 12 per cent cattle, 3 per cent pigs)
Suspected source of infection	Infected frozen lamb imported from Argentina.	Infected imported animal products.

	1967-68 epidemic	2001 epidemic
Cause of spread	Mainly airborne, with relative humidity and wind speed and direction assisting spread. Cattle were the main species affected by disease. From mid-February 1968 there were 18 cases of re-infection on farms which had restocked. In 12 of these, recrudescence arose from incomplete cleansing and disinfecting of farms.	Initially, by movements of infected animals, particularly sheep, in which the virus was present but clinical signs had not been detected. Later by local spread, including through persons, machinery and vehicles that had been in contact with infected animals and where compliance with biosecurity measures had not been effective.
Cost to the Department	Around £370 million at 2001 prices, including £280 million paid out to farmers in compensation.	Over £3 billion, including £1.2 billion paid to farmers in compensation.
Introduction of national movement ban	After around a week, movement restrictions were extended to the counties adjacent to the Infected Areas to form a barrier zone and on 18 November 1967, 24 days into the epidemic, a Controlled Area (including national movement restrictions) was imposed across England and Wales. On 25 November, it was extended to Scotland.	A national movement ban was introduced just under three days after the first case had been officially confirmed.
State of United Kingdom livestock industry	Smaller and more compact farms. Fewer animal movements. Beef and sheep production more extensive, with the average number of livestock per holding less than half that in 2001. Movement of animals highly seasonal. Far fewer animals and much smaller land mass affected than in 2001.	Farm sizes and stock numbers have increased significantly since 1967-68, production cycles are shorter and seasonality has lessened. The livestock industry is more intensive and there are many more animal movements, particularly of sheep. As a result, the land mass of Great Britain affected and numbers of animals involved was considerably greater than in 1967-68, even though the number of cases was similar. While the cattle population had decreased by a quarter over the last 30 years to 9.5 million in Great Britain and the pig population by a half, to six million, the sheep population had grown by a half to 40 million in 2000, including 21 million breeding ewes. The sheep flock is the largest in the European Union.
Number of live auction markets in the United Kingdom	Over 800.	170
Number of slaughterhouses in the United Kingdom	Over 3,000.	Fewer than 500.
Numbers of veterinary surgeons	An additional 645 vets were mobilised.	Over 1,800 vets were deployed at the peak of the outbreak.
Number of days before military deployed	12	25, though the Department had been liaising with the military from day 1.
Number of troops deployed	400	More than 2,000 at the peak.

A1 **Areas infected, 1967-68 and 2001**

Infected premises by county - 1967/68 outbreak

Infected premises by county - 2001 outbreak

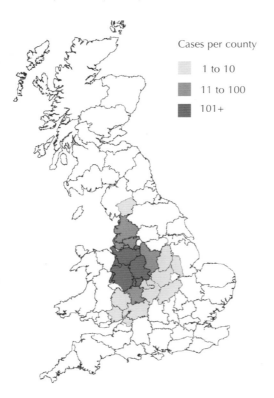

Cases per county

☐ 1 to 10

☐ 11 to 100

☐ 101+

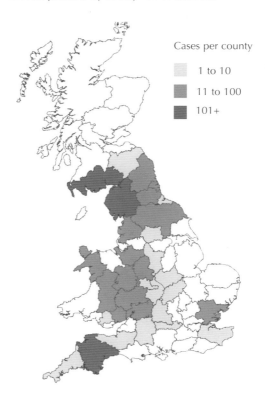

Cases per county

☐ 1 to 10

☐ 11 to 100

☐ 101+

Source: Department for the Environment, Food and Rural Affairs

A2 **Comparison of number of cases confirmed per week, 1967-68 and 2001**

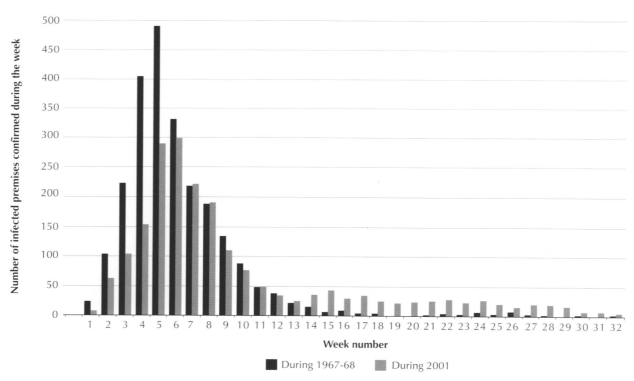

Week number

■ During 1967-68   ☐ During 2001

Source: National Audit Office, based on data from the Department for Environment, Food and Rural Affairs, for 2001 and the Report of the Committee of Inquiry on Foot-and-Mouth Disease 1968 (Northumberland Report), Part One, Figure III, for 1967-68.

Appendix 3   Study methods

Collection of information from the Department's headquarters

1. To establish a picture of the development of strategy and tactics, resource pressures and handling centrally of the crisis by the Departmental Emergency Control Centre and Joint Co-ordination Centre we:

   - interviewed key staff from the veterinary and policy wings of the Department and the Joint Co-ordination Centre. These included the Chief Veterinary Officer, the Director of the Joint Co-ordination Centre, heads of policy, epidemiology, veterinary resource and operations, foot and mouth disease communications, finance, procurement and internal audit sections, as well as staff from Joint Co-ordination Centre 'cells';

   - attended some 'birdtable' briefings at the Joint Co-ordination Centre;

   - looked at a wide range of files and papers, including the contingency plan, field instructions, daily reports by the Joint Co-ordination Centre to the Cabinet Office Briefing Room, daily situation reports sent in by Disease Control Centres, weekly epidemiology reports and papers covering development and implementation of the disease control strategy, resources and finance; and

   - analysed information held by the Department on expenditure, use of its websites and helplines and, to establish speed of slaughter and disposal over the crisis, data from the Disease Control System.

Visits to the Department's Disease Control Centres

2. Between September 2001 and January 2002, we visited local Disease Control Centres in Chelmsford (Essex), Exeter (Devon), Carlisle (Cumbria), Dumfries and Ayr (Dumfries and Galloway), Cardiff and Caernarfon (Wales) to establish how the disease control strategy was delivered locally. At each centre we:

   - interviewed those directing the disease control campaign locally, including the Regional Operations Director and Divisional Veterinary Manager, military officers, and more than 100 veterinary and administrative personnel from operational 'cells'. This included a focus group with temporary veterinary inspectors in Exeter;

   - met local stakeholders in Carlisle, Chelmsford and Exeter to obtain their views on how the crisis had been handled locally;

   - reviewed files, procedures and information management systems; and

   - visited mass disposal sites (Ash Moor, in Devon, and Great Orton, in Cumbria), operational rooms (including the Dumfries 'bunker') and an affected farm in North Wales.

3. Colleagues auditing the Department's Resource Accounts reviewed financial transactions in depth, including contracts and slaughter compensation payments.

Collection of information from other government departments, agencies and the devolved administrations

Cabinet Office

4. We interviewed officials from the Cabinet Office's Economic and Domestic Secretariat and Civil Contingencies Secretariat and the Office of Science and Technology. We also met Professor Roy Anderson, Dr Neil Ferguson and Dr Christl Donnelly of the Imperial College, London University modelling team. We looked at Cabinet Office Briefing Room papers, minutes of meetings of the Official Science Group and relevant papers published in scientific and veterinary journals by the modelling teams.

Ministry of Defence

5. We met officials from the Ministry of Defence and armed services officers at Disease Control Centres.

Devolved Administrations

6. We interviewed staff from the Scottish Executive's Environment and Rural Affairs Department, the Scottish Environment Protection Agency and the National Assembly for Wales' Agriculture Department and reviewed documents during our visits to Edinburgh and Cardiff.

Other government departments and bodies

7.   We met key staff of the Institute for Animal Health, Rural Payments Agency and Meat and Livestock Commission and obtained information about their activities during the epidemic. We also met officials from the Treasury's agriculture team and the Department for Culture, Media and Sport.

Obtaining information from stakeholders and others affected by the crisis

8.   As well as meeting stakeholders during visits to Carlisle, Chelmsford and Exeter, we wrote to industry bodies, trades unions, trade associations, relevant charities, relevant professional bodies, commerce and academia, to seek their opinions on how the crisis had been handled. We also wrote to relevant bodies in central and local government. A list of those organisations that responded is at Annex A.

9.   Through our website, we also invited views from anyone affected by the crisis and publicised this facility through the trade press. We received more than 50 submissions, including from affected farmers, rural businesses and Temporary Veterinary Inspectors.

International comparisons

10.   We collected information, through the Foreign and Commonwealth Office and the Chief Veterinary Officer, on levels of disease control preparedness in Australia, Canada, France, the Republic of Ireland, the Netherlands, New Zealand and Northern Ireland and actions taken during the 2001 outbreaks elsewhere in the European Union.

Evidence presented to Parliament, other inquiries and reports

11.   Our work was informed by:

   ■   evidence presented by Ministers and officials to Parliament, including to the House of Commons' Select Committees on the Environment, Food and Rural Affairs, Science and Technology, and Culture, Media and Sport;

   ■   evidence presented to the local inquiries in Devon and Northumberland, and to the Lessons Learned (Anderson) Inquiry; and

   ■   reports published on aspects of the crisis by the National Farmers' Unions of England and Wales and Scotland, the Countryside Agency, English Nature, the Environment Agency, the Farm Animal Welfare Council, the Local Government Network, the Department of Health and others.

Annex A to Appendix 3:

Organisations and individuals who responded to our invitation to comment on issues covered by our study

ADAS Consulting Limited
Brecon Beacons National Park
British Chambers of Commerce
British Goat Society

British Horse Society
British Hospitality Association
British Meat Federation

British Meat Manufacturers' Association
British Veterinary Association
Central Association of Agricultural Valuers

Central Science Laboratory
Cheviot Sheep Society
Compassion in World Farming
Council for the Protection of Rural England

Country Land and Business
 Association (CLA)
Countryside Alliance
Countryside Council for Wales
Crofters Commission
Cumbria Chamber of Commerce

Cumbria County Council

Cumbria Crisis Alliance

Dairy Industry Federation
Dumfries and Galloway Council

Dumfries and Galloway Farm Business
 Steering Group
Elm Farm Research Centre
English Heritage

English Nature
English Tourism Council
Environment Agency
Eville and Jones

Farm and Food Society
Farm Crisis Network
Farmers' Union of Wales

Food and Drink Federation
Friends of the Earth
George F White Chartered Surveyors,
 Agricultural Valuers and Estate Agents -
 Alnwick.
Gloucestershire County Council
Grundon (waste) Ltd
Hampshire County Council
Highlands and Islands Enterprise

Holstein UK & Ireland
 (cattle breeders society)
Humane Slaughter Association
Institute of Directors
Institute of Rural Studies,
 The University of Wales, Aberystwyth
Institute for Animal Health

International Meat Trade Association Inc

Kent Farmline

Lancashire County Council
Local Government Association

Local Authorities Coordinators of
 Regulatory Services (LACORS)
Master of Fox Hounds Association
Meat and Livestock Commission

Monmouthshire County Council
National Association of Agricultural
 Contractors
National Association of Farmers' Markets
National Beef Association

National Farmers' Union
 (England and Wales)
National Farmers' Union of Scotland
National Milk Records plc

National Office of Animal Health Limited
National Pig Association
National Trust

North Yorkshire County Council
Northumberland County Council
Powys County Council
Pygmy Goat Club

Ramblers' Association
Rare Breeds Survival Trust
Royal Agricultural Society of England
Royal Association of British Dairy Farmers
Royal Highland Agricultural Society of
 Scotland (Royal Highland Centre)
Royal Society for the Prevention of Cruelty
 to Animals
Rural Centre, West Mains (Institute of
 Auctioneers and Appraisers in Scotland)
Rural Stress Information Network/ Ruralnet
Rural Stress Support Network
 (Herefordshire and Shropshire)
Scottish Agricultural College, Veterinary

Science Division
Scottish Association of Meat Wholesalers
Scottish Borders Council

Scottish Crofting Foundation
Scottish Federation of Meat Traders
 Association
Scottish Landowners Federation
Scottish Society for the Prevention of
 Cruelty to Animals
Shropshire Chamber of Commerce
Small Business Service
South West of England Regional
 Development Agency
Staffordshire County Council
Tenant Farmers Association
Tesco Stores Limited

Trading Standards Institute
UK Agricultural Supply Trade Association
UK Renderers' Association
University of Plymouth, Seal-Hayne,
 Faculty of Land, Food and Leisure
University of Reading, Centre for
 Dairy Research
Veterinary Laboratories Agency
Wales Tourist Board
Welsh Local Government Association
West Devon Borough Council

West Gloucestershire Branch of the
 National Farmers' Union
West Midlands Regional Group of
 Chambers of Commerce
Women's Food and Farming Union
Youth Hostels Association
 (England and Wales)

We also received submissions from:

■ Livestock farmers from Cumbria, Devon, Essex, Forest of Dean, Gloucestershire, Leicestershire, Monmouthshire, north-west England, West Yorkshire, Wiltshire and York.

■ Vets and Temporary Veterinary Inspectors from Cumbria, Gloucester, Scotland, Shropshire and Worcester.

■ Members of the public and affected businesses in Cumbria, Durham and Wales.

■ Valuers and auctioneers from Leicestershire, Warwickshire and York.

■ Farmtalking.com.

Appendix 4 The three independent inquiries

Inquiry into the lessons to be learned from the foot and mouth disease outbreak of 2001	Scientific review by the Royal Society	Policy Commission on the Future of Farming and Food
Chair		
Dr Iain Anderson CBE, a former senior executive member of the Unilever Board and adviser to the Prime Minister on millennium compliance issues.	**Professor Sir Brian Follett** FRS, University of Oxford and former Vice Chancellor of the University of Warwick.	**Sir Don Curry**, a Northumberland farmer and former chair of the Meat and Livestock Commission.
Membership		
Dr Anderson, supported by a small secretariat drawn from across Government and including a secondee from private industry.	A committee of 15 further members, comprising veterinary scientists, virologists, epidemiologists and representatives of farming and consumer groups.	Nine other members, with experience of business, farming, consumer interests and environmental issues, supported by a secretariat based in the Cabinet Office.
Working methods		
■ Meetings with key individuals, including the Prime Minister, and organisations involved in handling the outbreak. ■ Visits to key regions affected by the outbreak to gather information at first-hand, meet stakeholders and hold open public meetings. ■ Visits to other European countries to talk to key stakeholders about how the associated outbreaks were handled. ■ Review of documents. ■ Invitations to people to submit comments.	■ Committee members formed sub-groups on: surveillance and diagnosis; prediction, prevention and epidemiology; and vaccination. ■ Meetings with key individuals and organisations, independent scientists and representatives of professional bodies, including the Chief Veterinary Officer, Government Chief Scientific Adviser, and University modelling teams. ■ Discussions with international experts and representatives of consumer and welfare groups. ■ Visits to Cumbria, Dumfries and Galloway and Wales. ■ Open invitations to people to submit views and detailed evidence.	■ Public meetings held in the English regions to discuss farming and food issues with local stakeholders. ■ Sector-specific events with stakeholders representing: the food industry; farmers; consumers; the environment; and food wholesalers and caterers. ■ Views solicited from individuals and stakeholder organisations on the issues being addressed: more than 1,000 responses were received.
Terms of reference		
'To make recommendations for the way in which the Government should handle any future major animal disease outbreak, in the light of the lessons identified from the handling of the 2001 foot and mouth disease outbreak in Great Britain'.	'To review scientific questions relating to the transmission, prevention and control of epidemic outbreaks of infectious disease in livestock in Great Britain, and to make recommendations by Summer 2002'.	'To advise the Government on how we can create a sustainable, competitive and diverse farming and food sector which contributes to a thriving and sustainable rural economy, advances environmental, economic, health and animal welfare goals, and is consistent with the Government's aims for CAP reform, enlargement of the EU and increased trade liberalisation'. [The Commission covered only England]

Inquiry into the lessons to be learned from the foot and mouth disease outbreak of 2001	Scientific review by the Royal Society	Policy Commission on the Future of Farming and Food
Issues investigated		
■ Adequacy of contingency plans ■ Effectiveness and timeliness of the Government's response. ■ Organisation, co-ordination and resourcing of the response. ■ Readiness of the farming industry. ■ Impact on the wider economy. ■ Vaccination (policy issues). ■ Alleviation of the economic, social and animal welfare impact. ■ Effectiveness of communication systems.	■ The research base for identifying present and future risks of disease. ■ Adequacy of early warning/horizon scanning arrangements. ■ Adequacy of preventive measures. ■ Availability, scientific efficacy and safety of current disease control technology (including vaccines). ■ Potential for enhanced use of quantitative epidemiological models in understanding and predicting the spread of disease and the impact of policy options. ■ Hazards to human health. ■ Ethical and/or financial constraints.	■ What should we expect of the countryside, farming and the food sector? ■ What is good about farming and the food sector at present and what are the problems? ■ What factors are driving these good and bad aspects? ■ What can be done to make things better in the short and medium to long term?
Timetable		
9 August 2001: Inquiry announced. **14 December 2001**: Formal start of Inquiry, including publication of Framework Document and launch of Inquiry website. **15 March 2002**: End of consultation period. **January-April 2002**: Regional visits and meetings. **April-May 2002**: Interviews. **July 2002**: Final report expected to be presented to the Prime Minister, the Secretary of State for the Environment, Food and Rural Affairs, and the devolved administrations in Scotland and Wales.	**9 August 2001**: Inquiry announced. **11 October 2001**: Call for detailed evidence. **November 2001**: Visits to Cumbria and Dumfries and Galloway. **30 November 2001**: Deadline for submissions. **12-13 December 2001**: Chairman attended EU International Conference on Foot and Mouth Disease in Brussels. **January-February 2002**: Meetings with international experts and interest groups. **July 2002**: The Inquiry expects to report and publish its findings and evidence.	**9 August 2001**: Inquiry announced. **25 September 2001**: Consultation document published. **29 January 2002**: The Commission reported to the Secretary of State for Environment, Food and Rural Affairs.

Inquiry into the lessons to be learned from the foot and mouth disease outbreak of 2001	Scientific review by the Royal Society	Policy Commission on the Future of Farming and Food
Recommendations		
Inquiry not yet completed.	Inquiry not yet completed.	The Commission's report contained over 100 recommendations for shaping change in the farming and food sector. Key measures called for included:
		■ Early, radical reform of the Common Agricultural Policy;
		■ Retargeting of public funds towards environmental and rural development goals instead of subsidising production;
		■ Measures to strengthen the food supply chain and promote collaboration among farmers;
		■ A new drive on research and technology transfer;
		■ Honest, straightforward food labelling;
		■ A comprehensive nutrition strategy;
		■ A new national champion for 'local food'; and
		■ Simpler, easy to use free advice services for farmers.
		Two recommendations related directly to control of livestock infectious diseases:
		■ "The Department for Environment, Food and Rural Affairs in consultation with the industry needs to devise and implement a comprehensive animal health strategy."
		■ 'Full electronic traceability of livestock should be achieved as soon as possible. The Department for Environment, Food and Rural Affairs and the industry need to put in place better systems to trace sheep and pigs if their movements entail anything more than one movement to slaughter, as well as enhancing the current system for cattle. This will reduce the remaining paper burden on livestock farmers, by allowing more electronic data transfer."

Appendix 5 The Outbreak in Scotland

	Scotland
Context 1. Size and importance of the livestock sector	Pre-outbreak: 9.2 million sheep, 2 million cattle, and 0.6 million pigs. Agriculture contributed 1.4 per cent of Scotland's gross domestic product in 2000, with the livestock sector's share 52 per cent.
Preparedness 2. Date local contingency plans last updated before the outbreak	Inverurie Animal Health Divisional Office in June 2000; Inverness in September 2000; Perth in January 2001; Ayr in February 2000; and Galashiels in August 2000.
3. Date of last simulation exercise	Local contingency plans were tested biennially by Animal Health Divisional Offices. The last exercise was held in Ayr in 1999.
4. Involvement of stakeholders	Local exercises involved local and headquarters' State Veterinary Service staff, Scottish Executive agricultural staff, local police, local authorities and Scottish Environment Protection Agency staff.
Course and extent of the outbreak 5. Date of confirmation of first case	1 March 2001, near Lockerbie in Dumfriesshire (reported by owner on 28 February 2001).
6. Date of confirmation of last case	30 May 2001 in Berwickshire
7. Duration of outbreak between first and last cases	90 days The peak of the epidemic was between 21 and 28 March 2001, when up to seven new cases were being reported daily.
8. Date declared free of the disease	11 September 2001
9. Epidemiological groups and seeding	Two-main groups: Dumfries and Galloway, with 177 infected premises; and the Scottish Borders, with 11 cases. The Dumfries and Galloway cases were a subset of the larger Cumbria cluster. Disease was seeded by movements of animals and persons to and from Longtown Market, Cumbria, prior to 23 February 2001. The Scottish Borders' cases were a subset of the Northumberland epidemiological group.
10. Number of infected premises	187
11. Number of dangerous contact premises slaughtered-out	1,445 (see note 1)
12. Number of animals slaughtered on infected premises	132,000 - 73 per cent sheep and 27 per cent cattle (see note 1).
13. Number of animals slaughtered on dangerous contact and slaughter on suspicion premises	624,000 - 90 per cent sheep, 9 per cent cattle and 1 per cent pigs. 77 per cent of these animals were slaughtered on premises non-contiguous to infected premises and 20 per cent on contiguous premises, and 3 per cent were 'slaughter on suspicion' cases.

	Scotland
14. Number of animals slaughtered for welfare reasons	307,000, including 188,000 'light lambs', 49,000 sheep, 59,000 pigs and 11,000 cattle.
15. Proportion of country under Infected Area restrictions at one time	10 per cent, concentrated in the south, with two-thirds of farms in Dumfries and Galloway being affected.
Handling the outbreak 16. Animal Health arrangements	Under the Scotland Act of 1998, legislation on all animal health matters has been devolved to the Scottish Parliament and policy development and implementation made the responsibility of Scottish Ministers. However, the State Veterinary Service, headed by the Chief Veterinary Officer, has been retained as a Britain-wide body. This was because it was recognised that animal diseases show no respect for constitutional or geographical boundaries and there would be advantages from sharing research, analytical and veterinary resources. Concordats between the Scottish Executive and the Department set out an agreed framework for co-operation. They specify that the Department pays the compensation for notifiable diseases such as foot and mouth, but that the Scottish Executive provides the administrative support staff in State Veterinary Service offices in Scotland. The Assistant Chief Veterinary Officer advises the Scottish Executive on animal health issues. The Scottish Executive's Environment and Rural Affairs Department advises Scottish Executive ministers on policy and implementation of policy. During the 2001 outbreak, Scottish Ministers were responsible for policy, but were party to Great Britain decisions taken on its handling and the scientific advice on which it was based. They operated within an agreed policy framework while taking account of local disease circumstances, Scottish topography and farming practices and the views of stakeholders. Consequently, there were some variations in the detailed implementation of Great Britain policy, for example in the movement licensing regime.
17. Organisational structure during the 2001 outbreak	On 28 February 2001, a Disease Control Centre was set up at the Ayr Animal Health Divisional Office. The Divisional Veterinary Manager led on dealing with infected premises, dangerous contacts, epidemiology and surveillance. A Forward Field Station was also set up in Dumfries, close to the focus of infection using existing offices and the Dumfries and Galloway Council Emergency Centre. It included representatives from the emergency services, local authorities and the main contractor, Barr Limited. On 26 March 2001, a tripartite Disease Strategy Group was set up in Edinburgh to have overall responsibility for management of the outbreak in Scotland. It comprised senior representatives from the Scottish Executive's Environment and Rural Affairs Department, the State Veterinary Service and the armed services and oversaw the strategy and resource allocation. It met twice daily, formalising the arrangements for daily meetings which had been in place since the start of the outbreak. On 30 March 2001, two days after the first case of disease was confirmed in the Scottish Borders, a Command and Control Centre was set up at Galashiels Animal Health Division Office.
18. Regional Operations Director: date of appointment and role	20 March 2001. Termed the 'Operations Co-ordinator', he was appointed by the Scottish Executive to ensure logistics were in place to support the State Veterinary Service in dealing with infected premises and dangerous contacts and to support the armed services in dealing with the contiguous cull and pre-emptive sheep cull. He also promoted liaison between the armed services and state vets and took a key role in overseeing the 3 kilometres and contiguous cull in Dumfries and Galloway and the Birkshaw Forest mass disposal operation.
19. Dates and scale of military involvement	Operational in Dumfries and Galloway from 23 March 2001. Troops were deployed to Dumfries from the 52nd Lowland Brigade, 51st Highland Brigade and, from 29 March 2001, the 22nd Royal Artillery. They organised the transportation and destruction of carcasses for the 3 kilometres and contiguous culls. On 11 April 2001, the armed services set up a second operational base, at Newton Stewart, to deal with the outbreak in the Machars zone. The number of soldiers deployed rose to a peak of around 470 in early April 2001.

	Scotland
20. Pre-outbreak veterinary and related resources	Ayr Animal Health Division had 10 state vets, six animal health officers and 14 administrative and support staff. At the start of the outbreak, several state vets were sent on 'detached duty' to fight the disease in England Galashiels had a complement of 8 state vets, 8 technical staff and 11.5 administrative staff.
21. Resources available at the height of the outbreak	In Dumfries and Galloway, peak staffing was in early May 2001. There were 180 vets, including 162 temporary veterinary inspectors, mainly drawn from Scottish private practices and agricultural colleges. There were also 62 animal health and field officers and 80 administrative and other support staff. Some 130 Dumfries and Galloway council staff supported the armed services and vets on a full-time basis. Galashiels had between 30-40 vets at the peak. Scotland was able to draw upon skilled Agricultural Officers from the Scottish Executive's Environment and Rural Affairs Department, who were accustomed to visiting farms, to work as field officers, for example serving 'Form D' notices and supervising preliminary cleansing and disinfecting of affected farms. The Scottish Department's agricultural staff, as opposed to local authorities, carried out movement licensing.
22. Proportion of infected premises that tested positive for the disease	66 per cent* * Based on results available for 169 infected premises
23. Features of disease control	From 17 March 2001, there was pre-emptive slaughter of livestock traced from Longtown Market in Cumbria, including around 570 sheep in the Inverness area. From 22 March 2001 there was a cull of more than 400,000 sheep within 3 kilometres of infected premises. The contiguous cull, introduced on 26 March 2002, was applied to all contiguous premises at the leading edge of the advancing epidemic. Farmers' unions were generally supportive of the contiguous and 3 kilometres culls and standards of bio-security by farmers were considered to be comparatively high. There were tight movement restrictions within the affected zone. There was early involvement of local authorities.
24. Proposals to vaccinate	In March and April 2001 vaccination was considered and contingency plans made but veterinary advice was that vaccination would not speed up eradication or prevent further incidence of disease and would take limited resources away from disease control operations. Vaccination did not have the support of the livestock industry and was not pursued.
25. Speed of slaughter on infected premises:	
▪ slaughtered-out within 24 hours of reported suspicions of disease	49 per cent (Great Britain 41 per cent)
▪ slaughtered-out in more than 24 but less than 36 hours	33 per cent (Great Britain 32 per cent)
▪ slaughtered-out in more than 36 but less than 48 hours	3 per cent (Great Britain 6 per cent)
▪ slaughtered-out in more than 48 hours	14 per cent (Great Britain 22 per cent) *Based on data from 69 infected premises with full report and slaughter times available on the Disease Control System. The remaining premises did not have hours given for the reports of disease, but, from the dates given for report and slaughter, in only around 40 per cent of these other cases was slaughter likely to have been achieved within 24 hours.*

	Scotland
26. Speed of slaughter on dangerous contact premises:	
■ slaughtered-out within 48 hours of confirmation of related infected premises	14 per cent (Great Britain 32 per cent)
■ slaughtered-out in more than 48 but less than 72 hours	13 per cent (Great Britain 14 per cent)
■ slaughtered-out in more than 72 hours	73 per cent (Great Britain 54 per cent)
	Based on data from 862 dangerous contact premises with full report and slaughter times available on the Disease Control System.
27. Carcass disposal	Around 98 per cent of carcasses from infected premises were disposed of by on-farm burns, the remaining two per cent, comprising older cattle, were rendered in Motherwell. Around 1,400 sheep were buried on-farm, following a Scottish Environment Protection Agency site assessment. Greater on-farm burial was not possible because of thin soil and highly vulnerable aquifers (bodies of underground water) in the parts of Dumfries and Galloway affected by the outbreak. The Agency's policy was to consider carcass burial on a site-specific basis and to permit burial only where environmental conditions were acceptable and the relevant code of good agricultural practice could be met. The Agency advised against the use of certain materials on pyres, such as tyres, plastic materials or treated timber. The Fire Service advised on pyre construction.

For the 3 kilometres and contiguous culls the Birkshaw Forest mass burial site was used extensively from 29 March 2001. More than seventy per cent of non-infected premises carcasses were buried at Birkshaw. A further six per cent were rendered and 22 per cent burned. Before late April 2001, there were mass continuous burns at Hoddam quarry and East Riggs (on Ministry of Defence land), for Dumfries and Galloway, and Crook Knowes, near Jedburgh, for the Scottish Borders. Ash from the pyres has been buried in landfill sites and the impact on groundwater quality continues to be monitored.

Four Scottish slaughterhouses were contracted for disposal for the Livestock Welfare (Disposal) Scheme. |
28. Speed of disposal on infected premises:	
■ disposed of within 24 hours of slaughter	29 per cent (Great Britain 44 per cent)
■ in more than 24 but less than 48 hours	42 per cent (Great Britain 13 per cent)
■ in more than 48 hours	29 per cent (Great Britain 43 per cent)
	Based on data from 142 infected premises with slaughter and disposal times available on the Disease Control System.
29. Speed of disposal on dangerous contact premises:	
■ disposed of within 24 hours of slaughter	88 per cent (Great Britain 71 per cent)
■ in more than 24 but less than 48 hours	9 per cent (Great Britain 9 per cent)
■ in more than 48 hours	3 per cent (Great Britain 20 per cent)
	Based on data from 1,328 dangerous contact premises with slaughter and disposal times available on the Disease Control System.

	Scotland	
30. External communications:	On 2 March 2001, Scottish Executive and Dumfries and Galloway helplines were set up for foot and mouth disease queries. Information was also provided on the Scottish Executive's website. Information letters were sent out by the Scottish Executive's Environment and Rural Affairs Department to livestock farmers. Regular stakeholder meetings were held in Edinburgh and Dumfries. The National Farmers' Union of Scotland also played an important role in disseminating information.	
Costs		
31. Cost to the Department	£334 million	
32. Average farm cleansing and disinfecting projected costs	£39,000 per farm in Dumfries and Galloway (Great Britain £35,600 per farm) (see note 2)	
33. Valuers' fees	In England and Wales the Department reached an agreement with the Central Association of Agricultural Valuers that valuers should be paid on the basis of one per cent of stock value up to a maximum of £1,500 per day. However the Association did not represent valuers in Scotland where the Institute of Auctioneers and Appraisers in Scotland was the main representative body. The Department intended that the same arrangements for paying valuers should be in place in Scotland. However, the Ayr Disease Control Centre informed the Institute and firms of valuers that the fee to be paid would be based on one per cent of the total valuation with a minimum fee of £500 per valuation and a maximum of £1,500 per valuation. Thus they were told that the minimum and maximum amounts would be on the basis of each valuation and not for each day. As a consequence there have been a number of disputes between the Department and valuers over payment. Valuers are claiming some £700,000 more than the Department believes they are entitled to.	
34. Uncompensated costs estimated by the Department to: ■ Agricultural producers ■ Food chain industries	 £60 million £25 million	
35. Footpath closure and re-opening	Similar experiences to rest of Great Britain. Footpaths closed on 27 February 2001, following an Order made in the Scottish Parliament allowing local authorities and animal health inspectors to prevent access to footpaths and other land. From early March 2001 a risk assessment approach was adopted but there was genuine concern about the spread of the disease and footpaths only gradually reopened. On 23 March 2001 a model risk assessment was launched and a Comeback Code distributed. The Code was produced by Scottish Natural Heritage on behalf of the Executive. On 15 May 2001 guidance was sent to local authorities in Provisional Free Areas stipulating that footpaths could only be closed if supported by a risk assessment that satisfied the Department. On 24 May 2001, this access guidance was extended to all of Scotland except the Infected Area. By the end of June 2001, most local authorities had re-opened their rights of way.	

NOTES:

1. Data on animals slaughtered and numbers of infected premises are based on the Department's information. There are some small differences compared with the figures that have been presented by the Scottish Executive.

2. Cleansing and disinfecting costs are based on costs in October 2001. The Department is updating the figures.

Appendix 6 The Outbreak in Wales

	Wales
Context 1. Size and importance of the livestock sector	Pre-outbreak: 11.5 million sheep, 1.3 million cattle, and 0.1 million pigs. Agriculture contributed 1.4 per of Wales' gross domestic product in 2000, with the livestock sector's share 59 per cent. Exports accounted for 40 per cent of Welsh lamb and sheep production.
Preparedness 2. Date local contingency plans last updated before the outbreak	Caernarfon Animal Health Divisional Office in July 2000; Cardiff in June 2000 and Carmarthen in August 2000.
3. Date of last simulation exercise	No recent test of the local contingency plan had been held, although one was being planned when the outbreak of Classical Swine Fever occurred in East Anglia in late 2000, followed by foot and mouth disease in February 2001. Because staff in Wales had been highly trained in preparation for impending disease control exercises, they were used in the Classical Swine Fever outbreak in East Anglia. The remaining staff in Wales were rapidly overwhelmed when foot and mouth disease struck and consequently "the State Veterinary Service in Wales was not as prepared as it might have been to deal with an outbreak of foot and mouth disease" [National Assembly for Wales submission to Lessons Learned Inquiry].
4. Involvement of stakeholders	Discussions had been held with local authorities on their role in an outbreak and they were to be involved in the exercise planned. Whilst their role had not been explored in detail in the local contingency plan it was expected that it would have become clearer if the exercises had taken place.
Course and extent of the outbreak 5. Date of confirmation of first case	27 February 2001 at the Welsh Country Foods abattoir in Gaerwen, Anglesey (identified on 25 February 2001 by an official veterinary surgeon). The first case on the mainland was confirmed on 28 February 2001 at Knighton, Powys.
6. Date of confirmation of last case	12 August 2001 at Crickhowell, Powys. The last case on Anglesey was confirmed on 24 March 2001.
7. Duration of outbreak between first and last cases	166 days The outbreak in Wales was characterised by a succession of separate clusters of outbreaks with intervals between them.
8. Date declared free of the disease	4 December 2001. Anglesey was declared free of the disease in late August 2001.
9. Epidemiological groups and seeding	Four broad epidemiological groups: Anglesey (13 infected premises), north Powys (36 cases), south Powys (39 cases), and Welsh borders (including Monmouthshire and the Black Mountains) and South Wales Valleys (28 cases). In Anglesey, the disease was 'seeded' by infected animals brought from northern England to an abbattoir. In the mainland, the disease was brought to Welshpool market by a contaminated vehicle that had been to Longtown market in Cumbria. Further south, another cluster was seeded by visits to a Herefordshire dealer who had been at Longtown market. There was subsequent spread through movements of farm personnel and vehicles.

	Wales	
10. Number of infected premises	117 (see note 1)	
11. Number of dangerous contact premises slaughtered-out	713	
12. Number of animals slaughtered on infected premises	70,000 - 87 per cent sheep, 12 per cent cattle and 1 per cent pigs (see note 1).	
13. Number of animals slaughtered on dangerous contact and slaughter on suspicion premises	216,000 - 91 per cent sheep, 8 per cent cattle and 1 per cent pigs. 51 per cent of these animals were slaughtered on premises non-contiguous to infected premises and 42 per cent on contiguous premises, and 7 per cent were 'slaughter on suspicion' cases.	
14. Number of animals slaughtered for welfare reasons	833,000, including 595,000 sheep, 199,000 'light lambs', 34,000 cattle and 5,000 pigs.	
15. Proportion of country under Infected Area restrictions at one time	35 per cent.	
Handling the outbreak 16. Animal Health arrangements	Under the Animal Health 1981 all functions for dealing with foot and mouth disease rest with the Department since they were not devolved to the National Assembly for Wales in 1998. All employees of the State Veterinary Service in Wales report to the Department. Because of the legal requirement under the Animal Health Act 1981 for the Department and the National Assembly to implement legislation jointly in Wales, in practice the Department took decisions affecting Wales in consultation with the devolved administration. The National Assembly's Rural Affairs Minister took an active role during the crisis in presenting policies decided in London and answering questions in the Assembly. On 26 March 2001, the National Assembly was asked by the Department to establish an Operational Directorate on the lines of those set up in English Disease Control Centres, to support the State Veterinary Service. This was done under an agency agreement with the Department, under Section 41 of the Government of Wales Act. All expenditure on foot and mouth disease related issues came from the Department's vote.	
17. Organisational structure during the 2001 outbreak	Disease Control Centres were set up at the Animal Health Divisional Offices in Caernarfon (for Anglesey) and Cardiff (for eastern and south-central Wales). The Llandrindod Wells area office served as an outreach control centre for cases in Powys. It reported to Cardiff, but from mid-April 2001 was given greater autonomy and was headed by a temporary Divisional Veterinary Manager. For serological testing in the Brecon Beacons, a temporary field centre was later set up. From 26 March 2001, a strategic Operations Centre was set up in the National Assembly's emergency operations room in Cathays Park, Cardiff. A Regional Operations Director drawn from the Assembly's staff headed the Centre. It co-ordinated the foot and mouth disease operation in Wales and was tasked with ensuring a multi-agency approach. The Operations Centre comprised 15 staff from the National Assembly for Wales, who operated under an agency agreement with the Department, and a similar number from the State Veterinary Service, military, police, the Environment Agency and, from 9 April, local authorities. The two main private sector contractors (Greyhound and MDW Transport) also had a liaison point at the Operations Centre.	
18. Regional Operations Director: date of appointment and role	26 March 2001 The Regional Operations Director was a senior National Assembly official. He reported to the head of the Joint Co-ordinating Centre in the Department's headquarters, but operated under an understanding with the Department that he would consult and seek political guidance from Assembly Ministers.	

	Wales
19. Dates and scale of military involvement	Deployed from 26 March 2001. Soldiers from the 14 Signals Regiment were deployed in Anglesey, as well as Royal Air Force personnel. They became involved in unloading carcasses that it had been intended to burn on disused land adjacent to a RAF airfield at Mona. This plan was abandoned as a result of local opposition and successful negotiations on the availability of a suitable landfill site. On the mainland, troops came from 160 Brigade and the Household Cavalry and also included Gurkhas, who helped round up sheep in the Brecon Beacons. From mid-June 2001, the Household Cavalry were replaced by a small Territorial Army transport and logistics unit. At the height of the crisis more than 600 armed services personnel assisted, playing a key role in the logistics of slaughter and disposal, particularly for the contiguous cull.
20. Pre-outbreak veterinary and related resources	Cardiff Animal Health Division had eight full-time state veterinary officers: five at Cardiff and three at Llandrindod Wells. This was two below complement, but there were 2.5 temporary veterinary inspectors working on cattle tuberculosis cases. There were six animal health officers and 22 administrative staff. At the start of the outbreak, Cardiff Division lost three state vets on 'detached duty' to fight the disease in England, along with two animal health officers and some administrative staff. Caernarfon had four state vets (one below complement), along with the Divisional Veterinary Manager.
21. Resources available at the height of the outbreak	In Cardiff Division, there were 150 veterinary officers at the peak, chiefly temporary veterinary inspectors, recruited both locally and from overseas. Around 100 animal health officers and field staff, including staff from ADAS Consulting Ltd, and 200 administrative and other support staff were also involved. The latter included, in mid-April 2001, around 115 personnel provided by the National Assembly for Wales and administrative staff seconded from the Passport Agency. In Caernarfon there were up to 40 vets at the height of the local outbreak.
22. Proportion of infected premises that tested positive for the disease	59 per cent* * Based on results available for 103 infected premises
23. Features of disease control	In Anglesey there was a pre-emptive cull of 47,000 sheep in a 50 square mile area. On the mainland, the Chief Veterinary Officer made the decision that all sheep traded through Welshpool market on or after 19 February 2001 were to be culled. However in the light of a particular case, an infected premises at Llanfair Caereinion, where the tests came back negative, a decision was made to adjust the Welshpool cull to exclude lambs. There was intensive serological testing of sheep for understanding and control of the outbreak in the Brecon Beacons from June 2001, where risk of spread was increased by common grazing. A Movement Control Area was also introduced in the Brecon Beacons in July 2001 with local and long-distance movement licences revoked and intensified biosecurity monitoring. Bio-security standards among farmers were considered to be comparatively poor by the Department. This was partly a result of the structure and nature of livestock farming in some areas, with parcels of land held away from the home farm and movements of personnel to help out other farmers and for sheep shearing.
24. Proposals to vaccinate	In July and August 2001 the option of vaccinating all sheep in the Brecon Beacons National Park was discussed. The Cabinet Office Briefing Room advised against vaccination although agreed that Wales could adopt vaccination if the disease spread wider than anticipated. The vaccination option was not implemented as initial culling stamped out the disease.

	Wales
25. Speed of slaughter on infected premises:	
■ slaughtered-out within 24 hours of reported suspicions of disease	42 per cent (Great Britain 41 per cent)
■ slaughtered-out in more than 24 but less than 36 hours	23 per cent (Great Britain 32 per cent)
■ slaughtered-out in more than 36 but less than 48 hours	3 per cent (Great Britain 6 per cent)
■ slaughtered-out in more than 48 hours	31 per cent (Great Britain 22 per cent)
	Based on data from 99 infected premises with full report and slaughter times available on the Disease Control System.
26. Speed of slaughter on dangerous contact premises:	
■ slaughtered-out within 48 hours of confirmation of related infected premises	28 per cent (Great Britain 32 per cent)
■ slaughtered-out in more than 48 but less than 72 hours	10 per cent (Great Britain 14 per cent)
■ slaughtered-out in more than 72 hours	62 per cent (Great Britain 54 per cent)
	Based on data from 498 dangerous contact premises with full report and slaughter times available on the Disease Control System.
27. Carcass disposal	Around 62 per cent of carcasses from infected premises were burned on-farm, 35 per cent rendered and only two-per cent (chiefly sheep) were buried. The lack of clay and the reliance on private water supplies meant that on-farm burial was not normally an option. The National Assembly also stated that there should be no burial of cattle in Wales. Rendering was not used as much because of a lack of capacity and priority being given to Devon and Cumbria.
	Around a third of carcasses from non-infected premises were disposed of through burns, including mass burns at Eppynt, a further third by rendering and a quarter at landfill sites, including 43,000 sheep from the pre-emptive cull at the Penhesgyn landfill in Anglesey. A mobile air incinerator was used in the Welshpool area in May 2001. There were large public protests to the use of Eppynt, despite its remote location.
	Carcasses from the Livestock Welfare (Disposal) Scheme were disposed of mainly in landfill sites.
28. Speed of disposal on infected premises:	
■ disposed of within 24 hours of slaughter	62 per cent (Great Britain 44 per cent)
■ in more than 24 but less than 48 hours	12 per cent (Great Britain 13 per cent)
■ in more than 48 hours	26 per cent (Great Britain 43 per cent)
	Based on data from 108 infected premises with slaughter and disposal times available on the Disease Control System.
29. Speed of disposal on dangerous contact premises:	
■ disposed of within 24 hours of slaughter	78 per cent (Great Britain 71 per cent)
■ in more than 24 but less than 48 hours	8 per cent (Great Britain 9 per cent)
■ in more than 48 hours	14 per cent (Great Britain 20 per cent)
	Based on data from 710 dangerous contact premises with slaughter and disposal times available on the Disease Control System.

	Wales
30. External communications	The National Assembly set up helplines on 27 February 2001. Helplines were also set up later in Divisional Offices. Over 100,000 calls were taken by the helplines in Wales during the crisis. A communications strategy unique to Wales was implemented. This established 44 local public information points across Wales and a programme of mailshots to farmers on a variety of foot and mouth disease related issues (51 factsheets and 16 advisory letters were sent). Information was also provided on the Assembly's website. In Cardiff, from early on, Assembly Ministers gave regular briefing sessions with stakeholders and there were regular meetings with local authorities, farmers and farmers' unions. Senior officials also had many meetings with farmers to explain what was happening. In Caernarfon, there were daily liaison meetings with enforcement authorities and farmers' unions.
Costs 31. Cost to the Department	£102 million
32. Average farm cleansing and disinfecting projected costs	£44,000 per farm (Great Britain £35,600 per farm)[2]
33. Valuers' fees	Similar arrangements to England. The Department took the lead in dealing with this issue because of their legal functions under the Animal Health Act 1981.
34. Uncompensated costs estimated by the Department to: ■ Agricultural producers ■ Food chain industries	 £65 million £25 million
35. Footpath closure and re-opening	On 27 February 2001 an Order was made enabling local authorities to make blanket closures of footpaths. On 20 March 2001 the National Assembly for Wales issued guidance to local authorities and the public on what activities could be undertaken in the countryside without adding to the risks of spreading the disease. Guidance issued on 23 May 2001 encouraged local authorities to re-open all public footpaths, except those near infected premises. By the end of June 2001 most local authorities had re-opened their rights of way.

NOTES

1. Data on animals slaughtered and numbers of infected premises are based on the Department's information. There are some small differences compared with the figures that have been presented by National Assembly for Wales.

2 Cleansing and disinfecting costs are based on costs in October 2001. The Department is updating the figures and the cost for Wales is expected to fall to around £38,000.

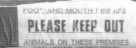

FOOT AND MOUTH DISEASE
PLEASE KEEP OUT
ANIMALS ON THESE PREMISES

ABN   ABN

⚠

DISEASE PRECAUTIONS
STRICTLY
NO ENTRY

Appendix 7
Disease control statistics by local disease control centre

Disease Control Centre	Affected Counties, Metropolitan Districts and Unitary Authorities covered	Number of confirmed cases (infected premises) (note 1)	Date of first confirmed case	Date of last confirmed case	
Carlisle	Cumbria	891	28-Feb-01	30-Sep-01	
Newcastle	Darlington; Durham; Newcastle-upon-Tyne; Northumberland; Stockton-on-Tees	190	23-Feb-01	29-Sep-01	
Ayr and Dumfries	Dumfries and Galloway	177	01-Mar-01	23-May-01	
Exeter	Devon	172	25-Feb-01	17-Jun-01	
Leeds	Bradford; Leeds; North Yorkshire	140	07-Mar-01	18-Aug-01	
Cardiff and Llandrindod Wells	Caerphilly; Monmouthshire; Newport; Neath Port Talbot; Powys; Rhondda, Cynon, Taff	101	28-Feb-01	12-Aug-01	
Gloucester	Bristol; Gloucestershire; South Gloucestershire; Wiltshire	85	26-Feb-01	17-Apr-01	
Worcester	Herefordshire; Shropshire; Telford and Wrekin; Worcestershire,	79	27-Feb-01	11-May-01	
Stafford	Cheshire; Derbyshire; Staffordshire	72	02-Mar-01	26-Jul-01	
Preston	Lancashire; Warrington; Wigan	55	27-Feb-01	17-Jul-01	
Caernarfon	Isle of Anglesey	13	27-Feb-01	24-Mar-01	
Galashiels	Scottish Borders	11	28-Mar-01	30-May-01	
Chelmsford	Essex; Greater London; Thurrock	11	20-Feb-01	12-Apr-01	
Taunton	Somerset	9	08-Mar-01	17-Jun-01	
Leicester	Leicestershire; Northamptonshire; Warwickshire	9	27-Feb-01	23-Apr-01	
Reigate	Kent; Medway	5	10-Mar-01	02-Apr-01	
Truro	Cornwall	4	02-Mar-01	06-Apr-01	
Reading	Oxfordshire	2	03-Mar-01	15-Mar-01	

NOTES

1. For certain local authority areas and counties, such as Cumbria, Devon and Dumfries and Galloway, there are small apparent differences between the number of infected premises shown here (for the relevant Disease Control Centre) and in paragraph 1.10. This is because, in a few cases, where an infected premises lay on the edge of a county the case was sometimes handled by a Disease Control Centre in a neighbouring county.

2. There were a further 51 state vets based at Animal Health Divisional Offices that did not have confirmed cases.

3. Based on analysis by the Department of data extracted from the Disease Control System in May 2002. The figures are for the period of the entire epidemic.

Source: the Department.

Days with the disease	Number of vets working on 10 April 2001 (note 2)	Per cent of confirmed cases which tested positive for the virus (note 3)	Per cent of infected premises slaughtered out within 24 hours of report (note 3)	Per cent of infected premises where disposal completed within 24 hours of slaughter (note 3)	Average number of dangerous contact premises for each infected premises	Per cent of dangerous contact premises slaughtered out within 48 hours (note 3)
214	243	89	33	38	3	53
218	71	74	20	53	3	27
83	61	65	27	51	7	9
112	332	69	26	9	5	12
164	28	93	57	77	5	38
165	38	59	37	65	4	24
50	66	31	33	41	3	15
73	39	36	38	8	5	5
146	51	47	45	57	2	3
140	35	85	39	92	4	24
25	24	45	27	17	17	0
63	29	82	38	91	6	26
51	16	91	10	30	1	0
101	8	89	60	89	5	24
55	19	71	13	25	4	0
23	13	40	0	0	4	0
35	24	50	0	0	6	50
12	4	100	0	50	2	0